Adam Hart-Davis
31 Berkeley Road
Bishopston
Bristol BS7 8HF

EDWARD JENNER'S COWPOX VACCINE : THE HISTORY OF A MEDICAL MYTH

Peter Razzell

Caliban Books

First published 1977 by

Caliban Books

13 The Dock, Firle, Sussex BN8 6NY

(Telephone Glynde 335)

ISBN 0 904573 02 8

Printed in Great Britain by

Newhaven Press, 44 Meeching Road, Newhaven, Sussex BN9 9RH

CONTENTS

CONTENTS

INTRODUCTION

The thesis propounded in this book is a controversial one: it is argued that the vaccines used by Edward Jenner, after his initial trial experiments with cowpox inoculation, were derived not from cowpox but from smallpox, and that the bulk of the vaccine used for the first forty years or so of the nineteenth century was an attenuated strain of smallpox virus. Given that the inoculation of smallpox virus had been successfully practised in England nearly eighty years before his first publication on cowpox inoculation, this conclusion substantially undermines the heroic role in which the history of medicine has cast Jenner, with its emphasis on the epoch-making quality of his discovery of the prophylactic powers of cowpox against smallpox.

In spite of the controversial nature of my argument, I have attempted to avoid a polemical tone and tried to present all the relevant evidence, even where it appears to go against my case. Hopefully, the abundance of historical literature for the many countries where the early vaccines were sent, which has not always been available to me, will enable a subsequent objective evaluation of my central hypothesis. I have resisted the temptation to avoid entering the specialised field of virology, in the belief that I owe the reader an opinion on the medical interpretation of the historical findings. I have greatly benefited from talking with Professor Keith Dumbell, Dr. Alan Downie and Derrick Baxby on this aspect of the work, but in spite of the virological complexities and possibilities revealed by this discussion, I have committed myself to the hypothesis which I think both fits the evidence and is plausible, in the belief that this will provoke further fruitful discussion and work.

I would like to thank Dr. Edwin Clarke, Director of the Wellcome Institute for the History of Medicine, who kindly read the manuscript of the book and has given me general encouragement, as well as the library staff of the Institute who were of great help. My final thanks are to the Wellcome Trust for the research fellowship which enabled me to take one year off from my regular teaching duties, and complete the work and write up the results of this book. Needless to say, all errors of interpretation and analysis are my sole responsibility.

Peter Razzell

Bedford College,

London, N.W.1.

CHAPTER 1

Jenner's Early Experience of Cowpox Inoculation

On December 11th, 1799, Dr. Andre of Petworth in Sussex, wrote the following account of the cowpox vaccine which had been sent to him for his practice of vaccination:

> "The matter sent from Brighton to Petworth produced a disease in every shape resembling smallpox: the time of sickening, the symptoms, the eruptions and their maturation were the same. The number inoculated was fourteen. Three of these were children at the breast; the number of eruptions in them was from three to twelve. The ages of the remaining eleven were from three to fourteen, and the numbers of eruptions from fifty to a thousand."[1]

An elderly woman visiting the house in which the children were isolated caught smallpox, infected her husband, and died soon afterwards of the disease.[2] The vaccination of the children had been sponsored by Lord Egremont, one of the most influential early supporters of vaccination, and as a result of this incident, he became highly anxious about the reliability and safety of the new practice. Jenner, writing to meet these anxieties, explained the origin of the contamination of the vaccine, which in the first instance had been supplied by Dr. George Pearson:

> "About a twelvemonth ago Dr. Woodville, physician to the Smallpox Hospital, procured some virus from a cow at one of the London milk farms, and inoculated with it several patients at the Smallpox Hospital. Fearful that the infection was not advancing properly in some of their arms he inoculated them (some on the third, others on the fifth day afterwards) with smallpox matter. Both inoculations took effect; and thus, in my opinion, a foundation was laid for much subsequent error and confusion . . . Dr. Pearson . . . was then, and had been, busily employed not only inoculating from this source, but in dispersing threads embued in the virus to various

> places in our own country, and to many parts of the Continent . . . In many places where the threads were sent a disease like mild smallpox frequently appeared; yet, curious to relate, the matter, after it had been used six or seven months, gave up the variolous character entirely and assumed the vaccine; the pustules declined more and more, and at length became extinct. I made a few experiments myself with this matter, and saw a few pustules on my first patients; but in my subsequent inoculations there were none."[3]

Jenner successfully convinced Lord Egremont and subsequent medical opinion that the problem of the contamination of vaccine was confined to that immediately deriving from the Woodville/Pearson lymph. Although he admitted to using it on an experimental basis, Jenner's letter implies that it did not form a main part of his own vaccine stock. I shall argue in this book, that **the bulk of the vaccine used by Jenner throughout his lifetime was the same as that which caused the smallpox outbreak at Petworth.** Evidence will be presented to show that Jenner's main stock of vaccine was derived from one of Woodville's patients who had about three hundred smallpox pustules and that this vaccine produced in the first year or so of its use cases of mild inoculated smallpox, and on at least one occasion, was probably responsible for starting a severe epidemic.

Jenner's first experiment in vaccination took place on the 14th May, 1796, when he inoculated James Phipps with cowpox taken from the hand of the milkmaid Sarah Nelmes, who lived in the neighbourhood of Berkeley. Phipps was subsequently variolated on the 1st July, and successfully resisted infection.[4] After this first trial vaccination, Jenner did not achieve further success until the spring of 1798, when more than thirteen people were vaccinated again with cowpox discovered in the Berkeley area.[5] (Some of these were vaccinated with lymph taken from the arms of those inoculated with primary cowpox — it should be remembered that until 1881 humanized lymph was the main source of smallpox vaccine in this country, and that it was only in the present century that calf lymph became the standard mode of transmission and preservation of vaccine). Jenner did not publish details of all these cases, but it appears that on three of them "an extensive erysipelatous inflammation . . . with some degree of pain" occurred, which was treated by the application of mercurial ointment.[6] In order to prevent a repetition of this complication, Jenner applied "a little mild caustic" to the vesicle at the site of the injection of two of the children vaccinated.[7] These reactions in the first series of vaccinations were sufficiently severe to lead Jenner to hesitate about the advisability of vaccinating very young children, for at the end of the original manuscript of the *Inquiry* he wrote, "How far it may be admissible on the tender skins of infants further experiments must determine."[8]

According to Baron, Jenner's biographer, he left Berkeley for London on the 24th April, 1798 and stayed there until the 14th July, unsuccessfully attempting to interest the medical profession in his discovery. He took lymph from one of his previously vaccinated patients in dried form, and after being unable to find patients in London to try it on, he left a supply with Cline at the end of July. Cline successfully vaccinated one person with this lymph, but failed to get it to take in three subsequent cases vaccinated.[9] With this failure Jenner appears to have lost the supply of vaccine (it is not clear whether he himself took some back with him to Berkeley, and failed to propagate it). After the initial set of successful cowpox inoculations, Jenner had a series of failures in the remaining months of 1798. In the following year he wrote:

> "Four or five servants were inoculated at a farm contiguous to this place, last summer, with matter taken from an infected cow. A little inflammation appeared on all their arms, but died away without producing a pustule; yet all these servants caught the disease within a month afterwards from milking the infected cows, and some of them had it severely . . . [later] The Cow Pox appeared at a farm in the village of Stonehouse, in this county, about Michaelmas last, and . . . out of six patients that I lately inoculated two of them only were infected."[10]

Both of the two children infected with the Stonehouse lymph had ulcerated and very sore arms, and in one of them Jenner was again forced to treat the vesicle with a special ointment preparation.[11] The results were sufficiently severe for him to recommend the use of caustic in such cases:

> "Although the application I have mentioned in the case of Mary Hearn proved sufficient to check the progress of ulceration and prevent any secondary symptoms, yet, after the pustule has exerted its influence, I should prefer the destroying it quickly and effectually to any other mode. The term caustic to a tender ear (and I conceive none will feel more interested in this Inquiry than the anxious guardians of a nursery) may sound harsh and unpleasing, but every solicitude that may arise on this account will no longer exist, when it is understood that the pustule in a state fit to be acted upon is then quite superficial, and that it does not occupy the space of a silver penny."[12]

Although Jenner tried to make light of the recommendation of caustic and the anxieties that parents might feel on this score, his colleagues Woodville and Pearson believed that he had underestimated the likely strength of parental reaction on what they felt was such a drastic procedure. Pearson wrote to Jenner on the 15th February, 1799:

> "On telling Dr. Woodville that I had been anxious about your publishing the use of caustic, he replied, 'that would damn the whole business.' Be assured that if the practice cannot be introduced without the caustic, or call it by any other name, it will never succeed with the public."[13]

Woodville and Pearson did not realise at this time that Jenner had experienced very severe reactions in his primary cowpox inoculations (which he did not publish) and this only came out subsequently through information published by other practitioners. Jenner had first used the Stonehouse lymph on the 2nd December, 1798, and eleven days later on the 13th, he had allowed a neighbouring surgeon, Mr. Darke, to take some for the vaccination of five patients living in

Stroud.[14] On three of these, there was only a slight inflammation of the arm and minor scabbing — and none of them resisted variolation on the eighth day after their vaccination.[15] On the two others, there was a sore and painful inflammation of the arm, the severity of the symptoms being disputed by the two independent accounts given of the events concerned, one claiming that they "suffered severely from violent inflammation and alarming ulcerations in their arms,"[16] the other that only on one of them was the inflammation "**troublesome** and **disagreeable,** but not . . . an **alarming** and **dreadful** circumstance".[17] Yet five years later, Mr. Henry Hicks, a friend and ardent supporter of Jenner's (he had been one of the first people to have his own children vaccinated) wrote of this incident:

> ". . . I have myself been a witness to many instances of very bad sore arms in the early part of the Vaccine practice; and the Rev. Mr. Colborne of Stroud, in this county, who had two of his children inoculated, was so much alarmed at the state of one of their arms, that further medical assistance was called in, and he declared to me, that he would never have another child inoculated with Cow-pock matter. This happened at a very early period, and long before either Drs. Woodville or Pearson had interested themselves concerning it."[18]

The severity of the reaction on the arm was not the only problem that Jenner faced at this time. He had failed successfully to infect the "four or five servants" through primary cowpox inoculation during the summer of 1798, and had only effectively propagated the disease in two of the six people vaccinated with the Stonehouse lymph in December of the same year — and these had ulcerated and inflamed sore arms. Darke, who had used a supply of Jenner's Stonehouse lymph, had an almost identical experience, only being able to successfully infect two out of five, both of whom suffered from sore and painfully inflamed arms. And to complete Jenner's problems, an attempt by another surgeon also living in Stroud — Mr. Thornton — to inoculate a Mr. Stanton and his four children with the Stonehouse lymph taken independently on the 1st December, appears to have failed in every case.[19] It is not therefore surprising that although Jenner had used the Stonehouse lymph as late as about the middle of December, he abandoned it (without ever stating why), and was unable to supply other medical practitioners with vaccine until after he had himself been supplied by Woodville in February, 1799.

One of the problems in assessing the early evidence on vaccination is the tendency that Jenner had of omitting details of failures that he was experiencing. For example, in a letter to Woodville at the end of January, 1799, he wrote that the difficulties he had with the Stonehouse matter had "not happened so generally"[20] — yet we know from evidence already considered, that there were more failures than successes up to this date. Two months later he himself admitted, "I have often been foiled in my endeavours to communicate the Cow Pox by inoculation."[21] It is likely that there were cases of failure not mentioned except indirectly; although he implied in the *Inquiry* that there were no outbreaks of cowpox in 1797[22] (Baron, later explicitly stated that cowpox had disappeared from the dairies between the spring of 1796 and the spring of 1798[23]), in a publication at the end of 1799, Jenner referred to "matter with which my inoculations were conducted in the years 1797, 1798, 1799, was taken from different cows."[24]

It is now known that the inoculation of primary cowpox is very difficult to achieve, and that success is the exception rather than the rule. Estlin, who was concerned about the deteriorating quality of vaccine through arm-to-arm passage, made extensive enquiries, and engaged in a great deal of correspondence with people working on the problem of primary cowpox inoculation and came to the conclusion that "matter taken from the cow, and inserted into the human subject in the ordinary method with a lancet, seldom reproduces the disease."[25] A year or so later, at the end of the 1830s, this was confirmed by Ceely who undertook a series of detailed experiments, the conclusions of which were summarised as follows:

"1. More than half my attempts to vaccinate with primary

lymph [cowpox directly from a cow], taken from vesicles at a proper stage, and possessing all the characteristics of perfection, have entirely failed. The same individuals have immediately afterwards been successfully vaccinated with dry or liquid lymph which had been long current in man.

2. A small number, vaccinated from the same primary sources, afforded results in various degrees of imperfection . . . Nearly all these subjects have been successfully re-vaccinated with ordinary lymph, from periods of nine to eleven months . . .
3. A still smaller number, vaccinated from the same primary stocks, have furnished vesicles in the highest degree of beauty and perfection. But even in many of these there has been more or less delay in the full development of the vesicles; and in nearly all, the number of vesicles has seldom equalled one-half of the punctures.
4. Precisely similar phenomena of entire failure, imperfect or complete vaccination, with all their attendant circumstances, have followed the use of lymph from perfect casual vesicles on the hands of the milkers; and the like results have frequently attended the early removes of lymph from the most perfect primary vaccinations."[26]

Ceely also noted the initial severe reactions to those primary vaccinations that did take, and described them as follows:

". . . it too often happens, especially in subjects with thin and vascular skins, that the vesicles burst or are easily broken during the height or about the decline of the areola; and if the subject be of a strumous or erysipelatous diathesis, of full habit, and possess an irritable skin, secondary inflammation is set up and becomes more diffused and deeper seated, the corium is destroyed completely, and a slough of the subjacent tissue is soon manifest, the surrounding integuments are deeply indurated . . . All this mischief, however, generally soon subsides . . ."[27]

Other workers in this field, however, did not take such a sanguine view of these complications; for example, Bousquet, who was one of the first to inoculate primary cowpox after the Jennerian period, gave the following description of his initial work:

> "In my first trials with the new virus (cowpox taken from a milkmaid), I made, according to my custom, three punctures on each arm. I soon had to give up this practice. The intensity of the inflammation was sometimes so great that it spread over the entire arm as far as the glands of the axilla. M. Gasc cannot have forgotten a child who he had vaccinated and had the kindness to show me. The vesicles were enormous, the inflammation so violent that . . . The crusts, when they fell off, left ulcerations which were very slow to undergo cicatrisation. It was at this moment that I understood, for the first time, Jenner's anxieties."[28]

We see, therefore, that Jenner's experience with inoculating cowpox up to the end of 1798 was typical of what was to be found by later workers: frequent failures of the injection to take, and in those inoculations which were successful, occasional severe ulceration and inflammation of the arm.

CHAPTER 2

The Origin of Woodville's Lymph

By the end of 1798, Jenner had performed only about a dozen successful vaccinations, most of which had taken place in the spring of that year. Although several London physicians, including Woodville and Pearson, had approached him for vaccine, Jenner was unable to supply any because of the failure of the Stonehouse lymph and the unavailability of any other sources. Towards the end of January, 1799, an outbreak of cowpox was discovered at a London milk farm in Gray's Inn Lane, and Woodville, physician to the London Smallpox Hospital, was informed of this; on the 21st January, accompanied by Thomas Tanner, a veterinary student from Gloucestershire and a friend of Jenner's, he visited the farm. After Tanner confirmed that the disease was a genuine case of cowpox, Woodville inoculated six people with the virus, and two or three days later, inoculated eight other people with virus taken from the pustules of milkers, after comparing them with plates in Jenner's *Inquiry*.[29] This dual confirmation of the similarity between the Gray's Inn Lane strain of cowpox and that previously experienced by Jenner is important, and it makes it very unlikely that Woodville inadvertently introduced a very severe form of cowpox (there is some evidence, although of unknown reliability, that such severe strains did possibly exist[30]). It is conceivable that one of the milkers accidently lodged smallpox virus on the udders of the cows — it appears that smallpox virus can be passaged in this manner without loss of virulence[31] — although the similarity of the symptoms on the Gray's Inn Lane cows with those observed by Tanner and described by Jenner from their experience with Gloucestershire cowpox, again makes this unlikely. The most important evidence in support of this conclusion, however, is that Woodville experienced problems of contamination with all of the different number of early strains of cowpox that he introduced into the London Smallpox Hospital, where the bulk of his vaccinations took place.

This hospital treated cases of natural smallpox, as

well as practising the inoculation of smallpox (variolation). This fact alone, seriously complicates the problem of interpreting the results of these early trial vaccinations: some of the people attending the hospital for vaccination resorted to that measure only because of their previous contact with a case of natural smallpox, while others would be at risk from catching the natural disease through contact with patients and staff at the hospital. Woodville was aware of the latter risk, and in his report on the first 500 vaccinations, he wrote:

> "Among the patients inoculated for the Cow Pox during the first week in which I obtained the matter of this disease, several were so circumstanced as to be afterwards constantly exposed to the infection of Small Pox. Having no proof that the progress of the infection of the former would supersede that of the latter, I used the precaution to inoculate the patients with variolous matter on the fifth day after that taken from the cow had been inserted."[32]

Jenner appears to have been mistaken in his letter to Lord Egremont, when he claimed that Woodville variolated these early patients on account of being "fearful that the infection was not advancing properly in some of their arms." Woodville published detailed case studies of the first 200 people he vaccinated: of the initial ten cases inoculated with primary cowpox, only one had no reaction at the site of vaccination within the first five days. The latter was variolated on the third day; of the nine others, six were variolated on the fifth day, two on the eleventh day after vaccination and one not at all. Six of these first ten cases had pustular body eruptions strongly resembling smallpox. It is now known that a full antibody response takes about ten days, and as seven of these people had been variolated within five days, it is not surprising that some of them responded to their variolation. However, this could not explain all the events which took place; the one person not variolated at all (the third case) had a reaction almost identical to that of inoculated smallpox, finishing up with twenty-four smallpox-type pustules, and although a smallpox inoculation would take full effect within nine or ten days of a previous vaccination, its effect would be significantly modified. The Vaccine Pock Institution conducted a series of experiments on this subject and found that two days after vaccination, variolation produced only a local effect; previously Robert Willan had found that although there was a general pustular reaction within the first nine days, the pustules rarely maturated.[33] Also, even more difficult to explain, future cases vaccinated with material taken from the site of the vaccination of some of these first ten cases, had numerous pustular eruptions, in spite of not themselves being variolated within the first ten days or so. At the end of the series, **nearly two-thirds** of Woodville's first five hundred cases had had pustular eruptions other than at the site of the vaccination.

This experience was in total contradiction to Jenner's findings about the results of primary cowpox inoculation:

> "Inflamed spots . . . appear on different parts of the hands of the domestics employed in milking, and sometimes on the wrists, which quickly run on to suppuration . . . these superficial suppurations put on a circular form . . . The lips, nostrils, eyelids, and other parts of the body, are sometimes affected with sores; but these evidently arise from their being needlessly rubbed or scratched with the patient's infected fingers. No eruptions on the skin have followed the decline of the feverish symptoms in any instance that has come under my inspection, one only excepted, and in this case a very few appeared on the arms . . . in the Cow-Pox, no pustules appear . . ."[34]

Jenner's conclusion was based, however, on a very limited experience, and must be compared with that of Ceeley who had acquired by 1842 experience of thirteen primary cowpox vaccines (although seven of these were derived from inoculating cows with smallpox virus). Ceeley concluded from this experience "that we have no better standard of comparison of the local and constitutional symptoms of efficient vaccine than that originally furnished and so beautifully illustrated by Jenner."[35] He was of course referring to Jenner's *Inquiry*, published in the summer of 1798, before Jenner had received a stock of Woodville's lymph. Although Ceeley's own experience of cowpox inoculation indicated that in the main it led to a purely local reaction at the site of the injection as described by Jenner, he did note that with two of the vaccines derived from inoculating cows with smallpox, there were minor eruptions of a non-variolous character:

> "In no adults, except in the case of my assistant, Mr. Taylor, was there any attendant eruption; nor in any child the slightest approach to anything of a varioloid character. Roseola, stophulus, lichen, were the principal eruptions . . . but small **eruptive** supernumery vesicles were observed in several cases at the period of full development of the areolae, and within its sphere, when **points only** were used. In one case a vesicle appeared on the shoulder, and one on the neck. In two other cases two vesicles appeared on the abdomen, all during the early removes of both stocks of lymph."[36]

In his discussion of the inoculation of natural cowpox lymph, Ceeley did not specify the occurrence of such eruptive supernumery vesicles, although he did state that "roseola" and "lichen" occurred in some cases.[37] He did manage to produce supernumery vesicles with such lymph, but only by injecting massive doses of vaccine and mixing it with the blood from the site of the injection — and then the supernumery vesicles only arose where the mixture had dried, although "sometimes they will appear even two or three inches distant from the puncture, when the blood, mixed with the lymph, has trickled down and dried there."[38] By adopting this procedure he was able to produce fifty such vesicles in a total of one hundred and fifty cases, although apparently he was unable to produce eruptive vesicles.[39] It would appear therefore that genuine cowpox inoculation very rarely produced secondary eruptive pustules, and that Jenner was correct in the conclusions he reached in the *Inquiry* about this matter.

Woodville initially assumed that taking vaccine from the site of a primary cowpox inoculation, was valid, even if there were smallpox-type pustular eruptions on other parts of the body, on the grounds that vaccination would remain a purely local disease, unaffected by the process of variolation.[40] Willan's experiments appeared to confirm these assumptions: cases in which variolation followed vaccination within nine days produced both vaccine vesicles at the site of vaccination, and modified smallpox pustules at the site of variolation and elsewhere. Material taken from the vaccine vesicles produced a purely local reaction typical of classical vaccination, whereas virus taken from the smallpox pustules produced results identical to inoculated smallpox.[41] In Woodville's cases, however, lymph taken from the sites of primary cowpox inoculation produced numerous pustular eruptions on subsequent cases [42] suggesting that he had somehow contaminated these sites of cowpox inoculation with smallpox.

What was the source of this contamination? One explanation which was immediately suggested by contemporaries was that the lancets used for the primary vaccinations had been themselves contaminated. This was Woodville's own immediate suspicion, but he discounted this possibility in his first publication:

> ". . . when I first observed a pustular eruption on Buckland (case three), the occurrence being wholly unexpected, I was not without apprehension that the lancet that was employed in its inoculation might have had some particles of variolous matter adhering to it. But this suspicion was soon removed, for, upon enquiry, I found that all the lancets which I had used on the 21st January were then made use of for the first time since they had been ground at the cutler."[43]

This does not eliminate the possibility that the lancets were contaminated, as before they were reground they would have been used for variolation in the hospital, and may not have been cleaned sufficiently to remove all traces of smallpox virus. However, there are other reasons for believing Woodville was right when he discounted contaminated lancets as the explanation of the pustular eruptions. In a further report published in 1800, he stated:

> "At various times I procured the vaccine virus, as produced in different cows, and with it inoculated patients in

> the Hospital; but the effects of all the matter I tried were perfectly similar: and pustules proved to be no less frequently the consequence of these trials than of those made with the matter formerly employed."[44]

It is highly unlikely that after having been made aware of the possibility of contaminated lancets at the beginning of the series of trial vaccinations that Woodville would have subsequently used contaminated lancets in all of his trial primary cowpox inoculations. Also, the timing of the first cases in the series is strong evidence against the lancet contamination hypothesis. The relevant details of the six cases inoculated with primary cowpox in the first week who had pustular eruptions are as follows: Case Three: not variolated, 24 pustules, starting on the eleventh day after vaccination; Case Four: variolated twice "during the progress of the Cow Pox infection", five pustules appearing on the fifteenth day; Case Five: variolated on the third day after attempted vaccination, four pustules on seventeenth day; Case Six: variolated on the fifth day after vaccination, 170 pustules beginning to appear on the thirteenth day; Case Eight: variolated on the fifth day, 300 pustules starting on the fourteenth day; Case Nine: variolated on the fifth day, three pustules appearing on the twelfth day.[45] The average period for pustules to appear after variolation is about nine to ten days[46] (although as Woodville and others pointed out, "this frequently happens much sooner or later"[47]), whereas the average period after the attempted inoculation of cowpox when the pustules appeared in these six cases was fourteen days. Given that most of them were variolated on the fifth day, this suggests that the pustular eruptions were the result of the variolation and not of the primary cowpox inoculation, contaminated through lancets with smallpox matter on them.

The above conclusion still does not explain why subsequent vaccinations, using material from the sites of attempted primary cowpox inoculation, also produced smallpox pustular eruptions. None of these subsequent cases were variolated before the tenth day and not only this, the other experiments that Woodville conducted attempting to inoculate primary cowpox from other cows produced pustular eruptions, even though "no variolous matter was applied during the whole progress of the infection." It is probable that the solution to this problem is as follows: (1) all Woodville's cases were constantly subjected to exposure of smallpox virus, either directly through early variolation for the cases in the first week, or indirectly for the latter cases, through natural smallpox infection within the confines of the hospital; (2) as has been seen, it is very difficult to inoculate primary cowpox and the probability is that many of Woodville's primary vaccinations did not successfully take, but merely created abrasions and cuts on the skin, with a purely local inflammation; (3) Dixon in his recent textbook on smallpox, has pointed out that such abrasions and cuts make ideal sites for the development of smallpox infection, and has speculated on the possibility that some apparently successful vaccinations during smallpox epidemics may have been just such infection of skin abrasions and cuts with smallpox virus.[48] This argument is supported by contemporary evidence on cross-infection; for example, Ring quoted the following case involving one of Jenner's nephews: "He inoculated a person with vaccine matter, and also with variolous matter, at about two inches distance . . . In this patient to whom it [the matter from the vaccine vesicle] was immediately transferred, a local pustule was only excited; but in a subsequent one, the taint appeared, and an eruption of about 300 variolous pustules took place."[49] And similarly, Willan, in his discussion of the contamination of vaccine with smallpox virus pointed to experimental evidence along the same lines:

> "When variolous matter is inserted eight or ten days before Vaccine Inoculation, the fluid in the Vaccine Vesicle becomes purulent, or is mixed with pus, after the tenth day, and in this state, according to the observation of Mr. Wachsel [of the London Smallpox Hospital] it will sometimes communicate the Small-pox only, but not always in the mildest form."[50]

The smallpox infection in the above case took place some days before the attempted vaccination, but the principle is the same — the secondary infection of the site of the vaccine injection with smallpox virus.

Woodville's vaccine displayed virtually none of the qualities of cowpox vaccine as described by Jenner: it produced numerous pustular eruptions, it successfully infected all those inoculated with it, and as Woodville himself noted, it produced a very different local reaction to that described by Jenner:

> "We have been told that the Cow Pox has frequently produced erysipelatous inflammation and phagedenic ulceration; but the inoculated part has not ulcerated in any of the cases which have been under my care, nor have I observed inflammation to occasion any inconvenience, except in one instance . . ."[51]

There was also a difference in the colour of the tumour at the site of injection: Jenner had noted from his early cowpox inoculations that this was "a colour distantly approaching to blue", whereas Woodville claimed that this was "an appearance which the inoculated disease never assumes."[52]

On the 15th February, 1799, Pearson sent Jenner some of Woodville's lymph dried on a thread, enclosed in an accompanying letter. According to Woodville, "the matter sent was taken from the arm of Ann Bumpus, who had three hundred and ten pustules, all of which suppurated."[53] As I will be arguing later that this lymph was the source of Jenner's main stock of vaccine throughout the remainder of his lifetime, it is of some importance to discuss in detail the history of this particular strain, through an analysis of Woodville's case histories. This strain was one of the two that Woodville passaged by arm-to-arm inoculation to form the basis of what was to become known as the "world's lymph". The detailed discussion of this vaccine will illustrate the symptomatic nature of the cases involved, allowing the reader to judge for him or herself the quality of this part of the evidence.

The following is a tabular representation of the genealogy of the virus with which Ann Bumpus was inoculated; I have taken the series from the initial inoculation from the cow on the 21st January through all cases vaccinated to Bumpus and her contemporaries. The number of pustular eruptions are indicated in brackets following the names of the cases concerned, and the date of the inoculation is also indicated.[54]

Cow in Gray's Inn Lane

21st January
Jane Collingridge (170)

30th January
William Mundy (15)
Elizabeth George (530)
Sarah Butcher (0)
Thomas Dorset (0)

6th February
Thomas Slade (4) (from William Mundy)

16th February
James Tarrent (from Elizabeth George)
(Resisted infection)

6th February (from Sarah Butcher)
Frances Jewel (0)
Ann Bumpus (310)
Jane West (20)

8th February (from Sarah Butcher)
Sarah Hull (120)
William Hull (200)
Hannah Hull (8)

Woodville's description of the primary vaccination of Collingridge was as follows:

> "Jane Collingridge, a healthy active girl, seventeen years of age. **Third Day:** The inoculated part began to be elevated and inflamed. **Fifth Day:** It was vesicated, and attended with itching. She was inoculated with variolous matter in the right arm, the former [cowpox] inoculation having been in the left. **Eighth Day:** The whole tumour is much increased in all dimensions; its form is perfectly circular, and it appears of a lemon-coloured tint. She now complains of a stiffness across her arms, and of a pain in the left axilla; the puncture in the right arm begins to be elevated and inflamed. **Eleventh Day:** She complains of a headache and pains about the loins; the tumour produced by the Cow Pox matter is now more inflamed at the margin, which is beset with minute confluent pustules, the variolous tumour is also advanced to a state of vesti-

cation; and she reports that last night both axillae were painful. **Twelfth Day:** She continues indisposed; the tumour is surrounded by an extensive efflorescence; the variolous tumour is of a deeper red colour. **Thirteenth Day:** The Cow Pox tumour is subsiding and forming a scab; that of the Small Pox is efflorescent; her headache continues; pain in the right axilla; several pustules appear. **Fifteenth Day:** There are small pustules round the edges of the variolous tumour; more pustules appear scattered over the face, body and limbs. **Seventeenth Day:** The scab over the Cow Pox tumour is completely formed; at its edges however, a fluid is still visible; the variolous tumour is in a state of suppuration; she complains of a sore throat, the number of pustules is now from one to two hundred, in no respect different from variolous pustules of the mild sort. From this time both the tumours gradually healed, and the pustules dried at the usual time."[55]

There is no doubt from this account that Collingridge had been very effectively variolated with all the classical symptoms of a case of inoculated smallpox. The only question is the nature of what Woodville called the "cow pox tumour". It appears that on the eleventh day after attempted primary vaccination there was further infection of this site of injection, with additional inflammation and more pain in the axilla. The fact that Collingridge had had 170 pustules "in no respect different from variolous pustules of the mild sort", and that these pustules had maturated ("the pustules dried at the usual time") strongly suggests that the primary cowpox inoculation had not taken in such a way as to modify the effects of the subsequent variolation. It is difficult to resist the conclusion that the "cow-pox tumour" had in effect become a smallpox one through secondary infection.

Four people were vaccinated from Jane Collingridge on the 30th January (four days after she had been variolated): William Mundy, Elizabeth George, Sarah Butcher and Thomas Dorset. The following are extracts from the published case notes which are relevant to the present argument:

"William Mundy . . . **Fourteenth Day:** Several pustules

> appeared upon his neck and back, but disappeared in two or three days without suppurating.
>
> Elizabeth George . . . **Fifteenth Day** . . . some pustules appear on her face. **Sixteenth Day** . . . more pustules show themselves . . . **Eighteenth Day:** More pustules have appeared . . . **Twentieth Day:** the pustules are very sore, and in a purulent state; their number is five hundred and thirty . . .
>
> Sarah Butcher . . . **Fourteenth Day:** no eruption.
>
> Thomas Dorset . . . About the **Twelfth Day** this man had four or five pustular appearances which he called pocks, but they seemed to me more like common pimples than variolous pustules."[56]

All three cases where pustules or pustule-like pimples appeared, were variolated, but not until after the pustules had appeared, i.e., from the thirteenth day onwards. The pustules erupted a little later than might be expected, assuming that the vaccine being injected was smallpox virus,[57] but as has been previously pointed out, there is considerable variation around the average time of pustular eruption. It is interesting to note that Woodville discounted the pustule-like pimples of Thomas Dorset (in the summary return of symptoms, he listed him as having no pustules), a tendency to play down ambiguous symptoms which was typical during the period of early controversy about the nature of vaccines in use.

On the 6th February, Thomas Slade was inoculated from the arm of William Mundy:

> "**Eleventh Day** . . . three or four pustules appear; the tumour is bordered with small confluent vesicles . . . **Nineteenth Day** . . . The pustules do not suppurate and are receding. **Twenty-second Day** . . . He was inoculated with the matter of Small Pox, which produced a redness for two or three days and afterwards gradually disappeared."[58]

This case displayed all the symptoms of a mild form of inoculated smallpox — the timing of fever, the appearance of eruptions, etc., and this was a direct function of the ostensible vaccination, as explicit variolation did not take place until the twenty-second day. Ten days after the inoculation of Slade, James Tarrent was vaccinated from "a pustule upon Elizabeth George". This was the first example of what became fairly common in Woodville's early practice — taking vaccine from eruptive body pustules which were indistinguishable from those of inoculated smallpox. (Woodville at this time came to believe as a result of these trial vaccinations that inoculated cowpox was a pustular disease resembling in many respects classical variolation). There was no reaction to either the attempted vaccination or a subsequent variolation; Woodville considered "this man as one of the few whose constitutions cannot be affected by either the virus of the Cow Pox or the Small Pox."[59]

We can now return to the group of inoculations of which Ann Bumpus, the source of Jenner's vaccine, formed a part. On the 6th February, Frances Jewel, Ann Bumpus and Jane West were all injected with virus taken from the arm of Sarah Butcher, who had had no pustular eruptions herself, and had been directly vaccinated from Jane Collingridge. No pustules appeared on Frances Jewel, but on Jane West twenty-two pustules all of which suppurated, started to appear on the fifteenth day.[60] The following is a verbatim account of the inoculation of Ann Bumpus:

> "Ann Bumpus, aged twenty years, was inoculated February 6th with the matter of Cow Pox, taken from the arm of Sarah Butcher. The appearance of the inoculated part in this girl's arm corresponded in every respect with those stated in West's case. **Eighth Day:** She complained of headache. **Tenth Day:** Pain of the head and loins; shivering. **Eleventh Day:** Two or three pustules appear upon her face. **Thirteenth Day:** Pains continue; more pustules appear. **Fifteenth Day:** No complaint; the pustules were counted and found to be three hundred and ten, resembling those of Small Pox. **Seventeenth Day:** Complains of sore throat. **Nineteenth Day:** Pustules drying. **Twenty-second Day:** Inoculated with the matter of Small Pox, but no inflammation was produced by it."[61]

Given that all three hundred and ten of these pustules suppurated, Ann Bumpus must have been inoculated with smallpox and not cowpox vaccine on the 6th February, and therefore the virus taken from her arm to send to Jenner on the 15th February was a strain of smallpox virus. Two days after her vaccination, Sarah, William and Hannah Hull were inoculated with the same virus: all had pustular eruptions (120, 200 and 8 respectively), the timing of which were typical of classical variolation.[62]

Soon after these inoculations, Jenner received the thread from Pearson, and vaccinated several children with it. On the 13th March, 1799, he wrote the following letter to Pearson:

> ". . . Twelve patients have since been inoculated with matter produced by this virus. They all took the infection. This is the ninth day, and they appear a little ill — no eruptions yet. The character of the arm is just that of cow-pox, except that I do not see the disposition in the pustule to ulcerate as in some of the former cases . . ."[63]

Baron states that Jenner received Woodville's lymph from Pearson "in the early part of March",[64] but as the latter had sent it in the letter dated the 15th February and Jenner had vaccinated his nephew Stephen Jenner and the boy James Hill before inoculating eighteen other people with matter from Hill's arm,[65] it is likely that the first two vaccinations took place some time during the last week of February.

It should be remembered that these were, in effect, the first set of vaccinations that Jenner had successfully performed since the initial dozen or so cases in the spring of 1798; unlike the attempted primary cowpox inoculations of the summer and winter of 1798, this new series were successful in every case, and showed no signs of painful inflammation and ulceration of the arm. Although Jenner made the general claim that Woodville's lymph produced similar results to his previous vaccinations, the specific accounts of this new vaccine were very different. The only detailed case histories that he published were for the two children first inoculated with it:

"**Stephen Jenner,** three and a half years old . . . 8th [day-

Arm] increasing in elevation. A few spots now appear on each arm near the insertion of the inferior tendons of the biceps muscles. They are very small, and of a vivid red colour . . . 10th. The spots on the arms have disappeared, but there are three visible in the face. 11th. Two spots on the face are gone; the other barely perceptible. 13th. The pustule delineated in the second plate in the Treatise on the Variolae Vaccine, is a correct representation of that on the child's arm, as it appears at this time. 14th. Two fresh spots appear on the face . . . **James Hill**, four years old, was inoculated on the same day, and with part of the same matter which infected Stephen Jenner . . . 10th [day]. The vesicle more elevated than I have been accustomed to see it, and assuming more perfectly the variolous character than is common with the Cow Pox at this stage. 11th. Surrounded by an inflammatory redness, about the size of a shilling, studded over with minute vesicles . . ."[66]

Although Jenner referred here to the eruptions on his nephew as spots, in some later publications he described them as pustules which failed to maturate. The discussion of Jenner's experience of pustules resulting from the use of his vaccine will form a major part of this book and will be dealt with in a later section; for the moment it must be noted that the pustule-like spots on the first case and the nature of the tumour of the second, indicated the variolous origin of Jenner's supply of Woodville's lymph.

In addition to admitting that the new vaccine led to less elevation of the tumour, with further experience of Woodville's lymph, Jenner summarised the following additional differences:

"The principal variation perceptible to me in the action of the vaccine virus generated in London, from that produced in the country, was its proving more certainly infectious, and giving a less disposition in the arm to inflame. There also appears a greater elevation of the pustule above the surrounding skin. In my former Cases, the pustule produced by the insertion of the virus was more like one of

> those which are so thickly spread over the body in a bad kind of confluent Small Pox. This was more like a pustule of the distinct Small Pox, except that I saw no instance of pus being formed in it, the matter remaining limpid till the period of scabbing."[67]

Thus, Jenner's experience with Woodville's vaccine was very different from his own with cowpox vaccine. One of the most important aspects of this difference was the success of the former in infecting people through inoculation; Woodville stated that Jenner had written to him acknowledging that his lymph "had succeeded better than any of the vaccine matter which he [Jenner] had tried before."[68]

CHAPTER 3

The Source of Jenner's Vaccine

The success of the Woodville lymph is of great importance in understanding the history of Jenner's own use of vaccines. The certainty of infection, the absence of ulceration and painful inflammation of the arm, and the fact that it was the first stock of vaccine to be successfully propagated beyond a limited series of initial cases, were probably all factors in explaining Jenner's future practice in its use. This does not mean that he stopped looking for independent sources of vaccine at this time — in his letter to Pearson on the 13th March, 1799, he still expressed frustration at the absence of cow-pox in the countryside, with the exclamation that there was "No cow-pox yet in the country!"[69] With the vaccine that he had from Woodville, he inoculated twenty children in the Berkeley area[70] and in the same month of March allowed Dr. Marshall of Eastington to take matter from the arm of one of his patients. Between the 22nd March and the 26th April, Marshall inoculated 107 people with it[71] and it is probable that Jenner sent out this lymph to other practitioners at about the same time.[72] According to Baron on the 21st March, Jenner left Berkeley for London, to take up residence there so as to establish his claims and reap the benefits of being the discoverer of vaccination; he appears to have stayed there until the 14th June.[73]

Baron claimed that Jenner became preoccupied at this time with the problem of the contamination of Woodville's vaccine and as a result acquired a fresh source during the month of April:

> "As the events which occurred at the Small-Pox Hospital were so different from what he had experienced, he was very desirous of procuring fresh cow-pox virus from the country. For this purpose he sent to Gloucestershire; and by great exertions on the part of Mr. Robert Tanner, he procured some from North Nibley. A portion of this he gave to Mr. Knight on the 12th April."[74]

Baron does not explicitly state the year in which this occurred but placed the comment in a sequence which suggests he was referring to the year 1799. He was probably mistaken in this respect, and his specification of dates of events can be shown to be in error for this period. He stated that Jenner had left Gloucestershire on the 21st March, yet the latter had dedicated his second pamphlet from Berkeley on the 5th April. It is quite possible that Jenner was not even in London on the 12th April when he is supposed to have given Mr. Knight this vaccine. More importantly, neither Jenner, Ring, Pearson, nor Woodville, who all discussed the relationship between various vaccines during this early period, mentioned the North Nibley lymph. Jenner undoubtedly would have discussed it if it had been successful, because of his concern for the difference between London and country viruses; in his second pamphlet he claimed that "further experiments made in London with vaccine virus generated in the country, must finally throw light on what now certainly appears obscure and mysterious",[75] and as this was written at the beginning of April, 1799, he would have certainly referred to the North Nibley vaccine in his third pamphlet at the end of the year, if he had used it successfully in 1799. (He discussed in the third pamphlet the differences between London and country vaccines at some length.).

Baron, later in his biography, makes further reference to a vaccine which is probably the same as that above:

> "On the 12th April [1800] Dr. Jenner received, whilst in London, some matter which had been generated on the cow by inoculation with the virus of grease by Mr. T. Tanner. Some part of this matter he transmitted to Mr. Wachsel, of the Small-Pox Hospital."[76]

The date that Baron refers to in both the above accounts is the same — the 12th April — and in both cases the virus was procured via a member of the Tanner family. Thomas Tanner had been apprenticed to his uncle, Robert Tanner, a "cowleech" and farmer at Rockhampton in Gloucestershire, before studying in London under Mr. Coleman.[77] John Ring made several references to the vaccine sent by Thomas

Tanner to Jenner in 1800 but none to one in 1799.[78] It is, however, possible that Robert Tanner had sent cowpox virus to Jenner in the spring of 1799 which failed to take on inoculation, and that like earlier failures, Jenner simply failed to mention it in his published writings.

Baron may have been confused by the fact that Jenner did acquire a fresh source of vaccine in the spring of 1799 with the help of Thomas Tanner, but it came not from Gloucestershire, but from London:

> "One experiment, tending to elucidate the point under discussion [pustular eruptions with Woodville's London vaccine] I had myself an opportunity of instituting. On the supposition of its being possible that the cow which ranges over the fertile meadows in the vale of Gloucestershire, might generate a virus differing in some respects in its qualities from that produced by the animal artificially pampered for the production of milk for the metropolis, I procured, during my residence there in the spring, some Cow Pock virus from a cow at one of the London milk farms. (It was taken by Mr. Tanner, then a student at the Veterinary College, from a cow at Mr. Clark's farm at Kentish Town.). It was immediately conveyed into Gloucestershire to Dr. Marshall, who was then extensively engaged in the inoculation of the Cow Pox . . ."[79]

In a later letter to Ring, Jenner mentioned that this London outbreak of cowpox had occurred "some time in April",[80] but it must have been at the end of April, because Marshall in a letter to Jenner dated the 26th April, 1799, makes no mention of it and only discussed vaccinations made with it in a second letter dated 8th September.[81] Jenner was clearly concerned with the problem of explaining the pustular eruptions resulting from Woodville's lymph; that he could entertain what, in retrospect, can now be seen as a scientifically unfounded notion about the differences between London and Gloucestershire cowpox, only illustrates how confused he was at this time.

Although Jenner had by the end of April acquired an

additional source of vaccine to that which he had obtained from Woodville, it is important to realise that **he did not use it himself** in his London practice, but had sent it to Marshall in Gloucestershire for the experiment described above. He made a number of references in his letters and publications to the use of the Kentish Farm vaccine which allows us to trace its history. At the end of 1799, he wrote an account of developments between the spring and the end of the year, and in that publication quoted letters from Marshall to illustrate the effects of using the new vaccine. Unfortunately, he confused the issue by (inadvertently?) claiming that Marshall's first letter described the results of the Kentish Town lymph, when in fact at the time when it was written (26th April, 1799) Marshall was still exclusively using Woodville's vaccine.[82] In a second letter, dated the 8th September, Marshall did in a postscript mention the new vaccine and stated that he had inoculated 127 people with it.[83] Three weeks previous to this Jenner wrote to Ring (on the 16th August) and included an account of the Kentish Farm lymph:

> ". . . Some time in April the cow-pox appeared at one of the great milk farms in the neighbourhood of the town. With this virus several patients in the country were immediately inoculated . . the cases now amount to more than seventy."[84]

As we saw earlier, Jenner was living in London from April until the middle of June, and from the numbers mentioned by him and Marshall, it would appear that Jenner himself was not using this virus by the autumn of 1799. On the 27th November, Jenner wrote to De Carro with further mention of the lymph and stated that "upwards of two hundred Persons have been inoculated from this source."[85] The first explicit reference to Jenner using it himself occurred in his pamphlet written at the end of 1799:

> "I have myself inoculated a very considerable number from the matter produced by Dr. Marshall's patients, originating in the London cow . . . and have dispersed it among others . . . From this source, Mr. H. Jenner informs

me, he has inoculated above a hundred patients . . . Whether the nature of the virus will undergo any change from being farther removed from its original source, in passing successively from one person to another, time alone can determine. That which I am employing has been in use near eight months, and not the least change is perceptible in its mode of action either locally or constitutionally. There is therefore every reason to expect that its effect will remain unaltered, and that we shall not be under the necessity of seeking fresh supplies from the cow."[86]

In this passage, Jenner very clearly contrasts his limited use of the Kentish Farm lymph with that of his main stock which had "been in use near eight months". The date when Jenner wrote the pamphlet in question is unknown, but it must have been before the end of 1799 because he refers at the beginning to Woodville having started his work on vaccinations "in the early part of the present year".[87] According to Baron, he wrote a letter "in the early part of December" in which he referred to publishing an appendix attached to the new editions of his first two pamphlets.[88] This appendix was issued with a separate title but bound with his first two works, the whole having a dedication to the King and dated the 20th December, 1799.[89] Therefore, although it is not known when exactly this third pamphlet was written, the evidence considered suggests that it was in the November/December period, which counting back the eight months referred to by Jenner, takes the origin of the vaccine back to the spring of 1799.

The nature of this main stock of lymph is indicated in a letter written by Jenner to Ring on the 18th September, 1799. Ring had written previously to Jenner asking for a supply of vaccine, to which Jenner replied:

"When I had the pleasure of receiving your letter there was no cow-pox matter here in a fit state to send you. That which is enclosed was taken about four days ago . . . This matter is from the source mentioned at the conclusion of my second pamphlet. It has been passing from one patient to another for upwards of six months . . ."[90]

The matter referred to by Jenner at the end of his second pamphlet was that sent to him by Woodville in February and used by him at the beginning of March, i.e., "upwards of six months" counting back from the 18th September.[91] Fresh stocks of cowpox virus did not become available between September and the end of November, because Jenner in his letter of the 27th November to De Carro replied to a request for a fresh stock of cowpox directly from the cow by stating that "I should be extremely happy to furnish you with matter immediately from the Cow, but in this part of our Island I have not heard of the existence of the disease among Cattle for several months past . . ."[92] The language used at the end of the passage quoted from his third pamphlet — "That which I am now employing has been in use near eight months . . . and . . . we shall not be under the necessity of seeking fresh supplies from the cow" — suggests that by the end of 1799 Woodville's lymph had become the main, if not the sole, stock of Jenner's vaccine. In the letter that Jenner wrote to Lord Egremont in December, 1799, he stated that "500 people were inoculated from this source [the Kentish Farm strain]"[93] — the past tense suggesting the ending of the use of this experimental lymph. Taken in total, the evidence on the history of Jenner's vaccine in the year 1799 strongly points to the conclusion that his main stock was derived from Woodville's lymph, and more specifically from the arm of Ann Bumpus. Jenner claimed that this main stock had not undergone any changes in the eight-month period that he had used it, but we saw earlier how he veered between dismissing the eruptions on his earlier cases as mere pimples of no account and describing them as smallpox pustules which had been eliminated through arm-to-arm passage. Whatever the logic behind his reasoning, Jenner had reached the conclusion from his experience with Woodville's lymph over an eight-month period, that in future there would be no "necessity of seeking fresh supplies from the cow". At first sight, Jenner's reliance on Woodville's lymph as the basis of his main stock of vaccine appears surprising, but it is less so when it is remembered that he had suffered from numerous failures and severe reactions in his previous vaccinations, and that Woodville's lymph "had succeeded better than any of the vaccine matter which he had tried before." Also his very restricted experience of vaccination prior to his use of Woodville's lymph and the variolous nature of the latter, led him to become confused about the nature of cowpox inoculation and its typical effects. Like most of his contemporaries he had only a very limited understanding of the nature of infectious diseases; he explained the decline in the number of pustular cases among Woodville's patients, by arguing that:

> "The cow-pox then maintains its ground having nearly destroyed the co-operating effects of the small-pox. And this event gives strength to what I have from the commencement of my experiments imagined that the latter is a malignant variety of the former; the parental root being the cow-pox."[94]

This belief enabled him to continue to use Woodville's lymph, persuading himself that cowpox was reasserting itself over the contaminated intrusion of smallpox. The early failures and severe reactions of the vaccines used before 1799, and the anomalous and confusing results with later ones, led Jenner into a form of defensive conservatism, keeping to the use of the vaccine which had been so apparently successful. He increasingly referred in letters and publications to his "stock" of vaccine, as if it were a particularly prized possession, the quality of which was guaranteed by Jenner's own personal stamp of approval and usage.

This attitude was most clearly reflected in the writings of one of Jenner's most important early supporters, John Ring. Having been supplied by Jenner with the Woodville lymph in September, he was forced to approach Jenner twice further for new supplies, because of failures in inoculating the vaccine. In November, 1799, Jenner's friend Paytherus gave him a supply of Jenner's stock, which, as we shall see later, produced 150 smallpox pustules on one of the first five cases with which it was used and was, therefore, presumably a further supply of the Woodville strain. Ring wrote in about 1801 that, since November, 1799, "I have been so fortunate to preserve the valuable stock; and have been able to supply practitioners in most parts of the world."[95] However, he did receive an additional strain of vaccine in May, 1800, for he described how Jenner had sent him some of the lymph derived from Tanner's experiment with the inoculation of horsepox; Ring did not indicate how extensively this was used, but merely noted that:

> "Many of those who were inoculated with matter proceeding from this stock have been repeatedly subjected to the test of variolous contagion, but in vain . . . This [vaccine] proved equally efficacious with the matter I had before employed."[96]

There is evidence to believe, however, that Jenner continued his policy of relying on his original stock, and ignoring new sources of vaccine. He had been responsible for supplying Waterhouse in Boston, America, with vaccine in the early summer of 1800, and as will be seen later in detail, this produced frequent pustular eruptions and probably in one instance, led to a smallpox epidemic. Waterhouse wrote to Jenner asking for fresh supplies, requesting matter particularly "fresh from the cow", in the belief that the vaccine first sent to him had degenerated through arm-to-arm passage. In commenting on this, Ring indicated that this was neither "necessary nor practicable"[97] and Jenner himself wrote in a letter accompanying a fresh supply, that it was from the same source as the first and "from that stock I am using among all my patients here" — and concluded — "The whole is from my original stock."[98]

One factor which only became clear with a longer period of practice of vaccination was the very limited number of cases that Jenner was personally involved with. Being primarily a country doctor, he was faced with the problem of finding enough patients for continuous arm-to-arm inoculation; he was forced to make arrangements with colleagues such as Paytherus and Ring to keep up a supply of his own stock.

Waterhouse referred to this specifically, in stating that "Jenner himself informs me that he finds it needful to give and receive assistance in order to keep up the necessary supply of fresh virus for use."[99] By the beginning of 1807, Jenner had performed less than 6,000 inoculations,[100] an average of about two a day since the beginning of 1799. With such a limited series of cases, it was impossible for him to keep more than one strain of vaccine going, given his anxiety about preserving a distinctive stock of his own, which could be defined and perceived as authentic.

In 1802, a vaccine derived from cowpox discovered outside of England was for the first time imported into the country. Ring described this event in January, 1802:

> "Dr. Sacco, of Milan, has sent to Dr. Jenner some vaccine matter, originally procured from a cow in Lombardy. Some of this matter, with which I was favoured by Dr. Jenner, has excited the genuine pustule; and in my own practice, and in that of others, is now spreading the vaccine preventative in every direction . . . These are the first instance of the production of the vaccine pustule in England, by foreign matter."[101]

Although vaccine derived from Milan did become important in other parts of the world— including among the British settlements in India[102] — it appears again to have been only used on an experimental basis in England itself. The most important evidence of Jenner's continuing reliance on the original Woodville strain in the longer term, came out of the enquiry conducted by the Royal College of Physicians' Vaccination Committee in February, 1807. Jenner replied in answer to a question about the attenuation of vaccine through arm-to-arm passage, that "he now uses Matter which was taken from the Cow in 1799; he has since taken fresh Matter from the Cow, and cannot perceive the least Difference."[103] Presumably Jenner's reference to fresh matter from the cow refers to the Kentish Town vaccine, that derived from Tanner's equine lymph (which was inoculated on to a cow) in 1800, and Sacco's vaccine from Milan. There are no further references in the literature to other sources of vaccine until 1813; on the 23rd July of that year, Jenner wrote to James Moore, Director of the National Vaccine Establishment:

> "Mr. Melon, a surgeon of repute at Lichfield . . . has sent me some of his equine virus, which I have been using from arm-to-arm for these two months past . . ."[104]

This direct use of horse pox once again appears to have been tried by Jenner only on an experimental basis, for three years later, on the 5th March, 1816, he wrote to Moore:

> "I vaccinate the poor here weekly, and . . . to the best of my knowledge, the matter [used for vaccination] . . . was derived from a cow about sixteen years ago. If there were a real necessity for a renovation, I know not what we should do, for the precautions of the farmers with respect to their horses, have driven the cow-pox from their herds."[105]

Jenner believed that cowpox was derived from horse-pox, but the important point about this passage is that it indicates that his main stock of vaccine was still that derived from his original practice. He was, however, rather vague about the exact origin of his vaccine ("to the best of my knowledge"), and the statement that it was taken "about sixteen years ago" would indicate that it originated in 1800 — when we know from the evidence earlier discussed, that his main stock was started in 1799. Similarly, in a letter dated 26th January, 1818, Jenner stated that all the vaccine "they have now in use in America, has been passing there from arm-to-arm for nearly the fifth part of a century",[106] whereas as we shall see later, the first of the series of successful vaccination in that country did not take place until 1801. This discussion of the age of the vaccine in use arose through widespread anxiety about a very significant weakening of its potency and its power to protect against smallpox; although Jenner rejected in 1816 the growing criticism that the lymph was becoming weaker through arm-to-arm transmission, in the following year, he appears to have accepted the need for a new vaccine, for having acquired another source of equine lymph in the spring of 1817, he sent it to the National Vaccine Establishment, to Thompson in Edinburgh, to Baron, and to the Rev. Dr. Worthington in the United States.[107] Baron stated that Jenner supplied "many of his medical friends" and that "matter from this source was, I believe, very extensively diffused."[108] This is the only solid evidence of Jenner using on any scale a vaccine other than that derived from Woodville. However, the main reliance on his original stock does not appear to have been changed by the use of this new source, for the National Vaccine Establishment continued to use Jenner's old stock many years after his death. The reports of the National Vaccine Establishment suffered, like Jenner's late accounts of his vaccine, from minor historical inaccuracy; for example, in its annual report for the year 1838 (printed 11th April, 1838), it claimed that it was still using "matter originally collected by Dr. Jenner, 38 years ago",[109] whereas the report for 1840 stated that "the principal source of our supply . . . [is] the original virus furnished by Dr. Jenner, which has now passed happily through successive generations of subjects in the course of forty-three years."[110] Presumably the latter refers to Jenner's first experiment with the inoculation of cowpox in 1796, but as we have seen, this did not become a source of vaccine for Jenner's later work. What these statements do indicate is that Jenner's original main stock of vaccine continued to be used until at least the late 1830s, a conclusion confirmed by C. R. Aikin, who had, in the first instance, worked for the Jennerian Society and later became involved with the National Vaccine Establishment. In 1840, he wrote:

> "The Jennerian Society was established in 1803, and . . . I have a strong impression, almost amounting to certainty, that application was made to Dr. Jenner to furnish the first supply of virus . . . Though it would be absurd in me to assert that it had never been changed or renewed from the cow, I can only say that I have never heard of any such change, nor ever myself had an opportunity of using virus taken directly from the animal, which, I think, I should have done had it been within my reach."[111]

CHAPTER 4

The Nature of Woodville's Lymph

In order to understand the nature of Jenner's vaccine, it is necessary to review the evidence on the use of Woodville's lymph and how its characteristics changed over time with arm-to-arm inoculation. In his first publication,[112] Woodville gave details of 459 vaccinations performed at the London Smallpox Hospital; 64.5% (296) were listed as having pustular eruptions, and this is likely to be an understatement, as some cases (like Thomas Dorset's) had an eruption of pock-like pimples which were discounted by Woodville. There were a total of 35,730 pustules, an average of just under 78 pustules per person for the total 459 people in the sample. This can be compared with statistics of pustular eruptions given by William Watson for a series of variolations conducted over thirty years previously: of 74 people variolated, 62 (83.8%) had pustular eruptions, with a total of 2,362 pustules — an average of just under 32 per person for the whole sample.[113] Although there was a higher proportion of pustular eruptions in Watson's series, Woodville's had a much higher number of average pustules. There were two main strains in Woodville's series, that derived from Jane Collingridge and a slightly later strain which, in the first instance, had been derived from the inoculation of a cow with matter taken from one of the first ten cases (James Crouch) subjected to primary vaccination.[114] Of 225 cases in the Collingridge series, 157 (69.8%) had pustules as against 102 out of 212 (48.1%) in the Crouch one. At the end of the Collingridge series, all the cases were being vaccinated with lymph which at some stage had been taken from a body pustule rather than the local site of previous injection, whereas this appears not to have been the case with the Crouch strain. The first three people inoculated with the latter, however, had 300, 105 and 350 pustules (this was with lymph taken from Professor Coleman's cow) and so although we cannot be quite sure that it was a pure smallpox vaccine, the evidence points overwhelmingly to this conclusion (the Crouch strain was probably more attenuated through arm-to-arm passage, with fewer passes through body pustules). Woodville summarised his conclusions about the nature of cowpox inoculation at the end of his *Reports:*

> "We have been told that the Cow Pox tumour has frequently produced erysimelatous inflammation and phagedenic ulceration; but the inoculated part has not ulcerated in any of the cases which have been under my care, nor have I observed inflammation to occasion any inconvenience, except in one instance . . . But it must be acknowledged, that in several instances, the Cow Pox has proved a very serious disease. In three or four cases, out of five hundred, the patient has been in considerable danger, and one child, as I have already observed, actually died under the effects of the disease. Now, if it be admitted that, at an average, one of five hundred will die of the inoculated Cow Pox, I confess I should not be disposed to introduce this disease into the Inoculation Hospital, because out of the last five thousand cases of variolous inoculation the number of deaths has not exceeded the proportion of one in six hundred . . . One important advantage which the Cow Pox is supposed to have over the Small Pox is that the former is not a contagious disease, and not to be propagated by the effluvia of persons infected with it. This is certainly true when the disorder is confined to the inoculated part, but where it produces numerous pustules on the body the exhalations they send forth are capable of infecting others in the same manner as the Small Pox. Two instances of casual infection in this way have lately fallen under my observation . . ."[115]

The conclusion is irresistable: Woodville's first series of vaccinations were producing results nearly identical to classical Suttonian variolation — he was inoculating smallpox not cowpox virus.

However, the severity of the results of his inoculations declined with arm-to-arm passage **when virus was selected from sites of previous inoculations.** Woodville himself noted:

> "that the matter taken from the arm of a patient, in whom the disorder neither produced fever nor eruption . . . has much more commonly had the effect of exciting a milder disease than the matter of the pustules, or than that which was obtained from a patient who had the disease in a severe manner".[116]

From the detailed case histories published, it is possible to analyse the effects of injections using different sources of vaccine, and such an analysis leads to a more specific conclusion than that suggested by Woodville. The following is what emerges from a breakdown of three types of vaccine, classified according to their source of origin: (1) of 106 cases inoculated with vaccine taken from the site of injection on 19 patients with no pustular eruption, 63 had eruptions (59.4%) with an average of 94 pustules each; (2) of 61 people inoculated with vaccine taken from the pustules of 11 cases with eruptions, 57 had pustular eruptions (93.6%) with an average of 96 pustules each; (3) of 219 cases inoculated with vaccine taken from the site of a previous injection on 43 patients with pustular eruptions, 122 had eruptions (55.7%) with an average of 135 pustules each. The result that stands out from these figures is the significantly smaller proportion of pustular eruptions amongst cases inoculated with material selected from a site of previous injection, irrespective of whether the patients from which the virus was taken had pustules themselves or not. As a result of Woodville's general awareness of this result, he began to select for his inoculations "matter . . . from those only, in whom the disease proved to be very mild."[117] Although he did not explicitly state that he was taking material from the sites of previous injection, this must have become the case, for he stated to a House of Commons Committee on vaccination in March, 1802 (over three years after his initial trials) that vaccination was a non-pustular disease, i.e., should be confined to merely a vesicular reaction at the site of injection.[118] He wrote a letter to *The Medical and Physical Journal* on the 13th June, 1799 in which he summarised the position on the new results of using only material selected from "very mild" cases:

> "In my *Reports of Inoculation for the Cow-Pox*, published last month, it appears that more than one half of the patients had pustules; I have, however, observed that . . . the disease in its progress from patient to patient, has actually become much milder. For out of 310 cases of cowpox, which have been since under my care, only 39 had pustules that suppurated; viz, out of the first 100, 19 had pustules, out of the second 13, and out of the last 110, only 7 had pustules."[119]

A year later, in the summer of 1800, he confirmed this attenuation of the vaccine through arm-to-arm inoculation, stating that he then had experience of the vaccination of "about 2,000 persons" — and that in the London Smallpox Hospital, "the disease continues to occasionally produce pustules, though not more than in the proportion of three or four cases out of 100."[120] By the end of 1800, "the number of pustular cases under the vaccine inoculation in the hospital, has been even less than three or four out of a hundred,"[121] and in March, 1802, still using the same stock of vaccine, when asked by the House of Commons Committee whether vaccination produced pustular eruptions on the body, he replied:

> "I believe they never do over the whole body; I have seen in some instances a few pustules in the neighbourhood of the inoculated part, but these instances are very rare, one in five hundred."[122]

Woodville, like most of his contemporaries, significantly distorted his perception of the evidence to fit into his understanding of it; however, all accounts of the results of using his vaccine confirm that it was becoming milder-and-milder over time, and that by about 1802 it was probably the case that only local pustular eruptions occurred, and then only very rarely. (Adams did admit in 1807, that "in the Small Pox Hospital in a very few instances, small variolous pustules have appeared after the vaccine scab has formed,"[123] but this was probably due at this stage to prior natural smallpox infection.).

Woodville was faced with a considerable problem in explaining these results, for he had all along believed that he was inoculating cowpox, and never abandoned that belief. A year or so after his first series of vaccinations, he began to argue that the occurrence of pustular eruptions was due to the "variolous atmosphere" of the London Smallpox Hospital, and that many of the people vaccinated had been inadvertently infected with natural smallpox.[124] Two factors make this explanation unacceptable: (1) very few of the later vaccinations at the Hospital did result in pustular eruptions, in spite of also being exposed to natural smallpox infection; (2) most medical practitioners using Woodville's lymph outside of the Hospital did experience pustular eruptions. In fact, ironically, Woodville himself initially attempted to rebut Jenner's argument that the "town air" had somehow contaminated the vaccine, by describing cases of pustular eruptions outside of London:

> ". . . of the cases which I have stated, several were those of patients who were inoculated eight miles distance from London; yet those patients, in the proportion of about one in five, had an eruption. And at a small village, still further from London, eighteen persons were inoculated with similar Matter, in all of whom it produced pustules."[125]

He later attempted to explain the eruption of pustules in the first example with reference to a smallpox epidemic then occurring in the area; he failed to mention the embarrassing example of the one hundred per cent eruption in the second village.[126]

Woodville also later claimed that his private practice was free of the problem of pustular eruptions and stated that other practitioners using the vaccine had had similar favourable experiences. It is difficult to see how he was able to ignore the numerous accounts which appeared in contemporary medical journals, describing frequent cases of pustules and general body eruptions. Ring expressed his own surprise when reading Woodville's claim:

> "Having conceived an early prepossession in favour of vaccine inoculation, and anxiously sought for an opportunity of putting it into practice, I was much surprised, and discouraged, by the result of the two first cases [with

> Woodville's vaccine] where considerable eruptions resembling the small-pox, appeared, attended with the other characteristics of that disease . . . What was my surprise at reading this paragraph [of Woodville's, denying pustular eruptions outside of the hospital], when not only the medical and miscellaneous journals and magazines, but the weekly and daily prints, have noticed the circumstance of considerable pustular eruptions, produced by matter obtained from the Small-pox Hospital! When the pamphlets written on the Cow-pox alluded to that circumstance! and when it has long been a common topic of conversation, both in private companies, and at all the medical societies in London!"[127]

These reports were not confined to London: we shall see that virtually every area of Great Britain and each foreign country which used vaccine had a similar experience. In defence of Woodville, it might be said that with arm-to-arm inoculation of the vaccine, the pustular symptoms became more and more ambiguous, a phenomenon of some importance in understanding Jenner's own experience of Woodville's lymph, and the characteristics of his stock, particularly during the first two or three years of its use.

Woodville himself does not appear to have distributed vaccine but had a working arrangement with Pearson, whereby the former was primarily responsible for production and the latter for distribution. However, Pearson did discover a source of vaccine soon after Woodville had found cowpox in Gray's Inn Lane and in 1802, he gave the following account of the early history of his part in the development of Woodville's lymph:

> ". . . to . . . Dr. Woodville, information was communicated in January, 1799, that the Cowpox was epizootic in Gray's Inn Lane; and at the same time I received the agreeable intelligence that the disease was also raging in the largest stock of Cows on the New Road, near Paddington to which no one could gain admittance but myself. With vaccine matter procured from these sources, Dr. Woodville instituted the trials of the new inoculation in the

Smallpox Hospital; and I carried on mine in certain situations instead of the Smallpox [inoculation] . . ."[128]

Although Pearson claimed joint origin of the vaccine employed in the London Smallpox Hospital — elsewhere he referred to himself taking cowpox from "Mr. Willan's cows in Mary-le-bone fields" in February[129] — Woodville made no mention of the latter in his report on the first three months' experience with vaccination (he gave the exact source of all his vaccine for the first 459 cases) and it is likely that he used it along with other sources of cowpox on a purely experimental basis. Pearson later stated that he had used the New Road/Marylebone source of vaccine in his own private practice with some success, but he appears to have been forced by the scarcity of private patients, to resort to a use of Woodville's lymph:

> "The matter which had never been in the Small-pox Hospital and which I myself took from the cows at the cow stables above alluded to, **scarcely ever** afforded eruptions like the small-pox; but when I obtained matter to supply my correspondents in the country, not having enough of my own hand, but obtained it from the Small-pox Hospital, it frequently according to the reports of my correspondents, and in a few cases where I practised it myself, did produce such eruptions."[130]

Pearson sent Woodville's lymph out to more than 200 medical practitioners in the United Kingdom, with an accompanying letter dated the 12th March, 1799.[131] By this time, he seems to have been relying exclusively on Woodville for the source of his vaccine; the lymph that he had sent to Jenner in the middle of February had been from this source, and when Ring had asked him for a supply, "I was informed that what he brought with him came from Dr. Woodville; not being able to take sufficient from his own patients to supply the increasing demand."[132] Pearson later mentioned taking cowpox "from a cow in March (1799) last,"[133] but as this gave rise to pustular eruptions and contradicted his other statements about the origin of his vaccine, he was almost certainly in error in mentioning this date. At the beginning of 1800 he summarised the history of Woodville's vaccine during the previous year:

> "In the months of January and February, 1799, the breaking out of the Cow-pock in two milk farms near London, furnished the vaccine poison which Dr. Woodville and myself disseminated, not only throughout this island, but also over a greater part of the continent, as well as to other quarters of the globe . . ."[134]

Pearson was initially very surprised at the results of using Woodville's lymph: "To my astonishment the disorder proceeded exactly as the inoculated smallpox."[135] In the letter sent to the 200 medical practitioners, he stated that "the whole amount of the constitutional illness [with vaccination] seemed to be as great as in the same number of patients in the inoculated smallpox."[136] Like Woodville, however, he soon experienced a decline in the severity of symptoms with arm-to-arm inoculation of the vaccine, and in August, 1799, published the following:

> "I must correct my statement of March last . . . Since that Report, or at least for the last four months, as far as I observed and been able to learn from others, the whole amount of the constitutional illness was not one half of the whole amount in an equal number of patients inoculated for the Smallpox . . . In my private practice, not a single case with eruptions resembling the Smallpox has occurred these last four months, and but a small proportion with any eruptions of other kinds. From my correspondents I have not had a single case of eruptions like the variolous since that of Dr. Redfearn's of Lynn [in April, 1799] . . ."[137]

With the decline of the severity of symptoms, Pearson, like Woodville and Jenner, began to deny that the vaccine that he was using gave rise to pustules and other symptoms of inoculated smallpox. He was soon forced to retract this belief because of the resurgence of virulence experienced with the vaccine used at Petworth. In the light of this experience, Pearson rewrote the history of his use of vaccine which is worth quoting at length because of the light that it sheds on both the changes that were brought about by arm-to-arm inoculation and (as we shall see later), the nature of Jenner's stock of vaccine. In February, 1800, Pearson published the following statement:

> "In the course of my practice, the latter end of February and in March following, I distinctly recollect four cases, in which I first saw eruptions from the vaccine inoculation, resembling so much those of the small-pox, that I should not have hesitated to consider them as belonging to this disease, if I had not excited them by a different poison from the variolous. I observed, however, at that time, some appearance of these eruptions different from those which usually occur in the small-pox. Almost all these eruptions, in the stage of dessication, afforded shining, smooth, black, or reddish-brown scabs; very few of them having previously suppurated. Finding, in several instances, that the matter from the inoculated pustule of these patients produced a similar eruptive disorder . . . I, from that time, avoided using matter from the cases in which such eruptions appeared. After this precaution, no eruptive cases resembling the small-pox, but certainly eruptions, in number from a single one to about a dozen, which were large, red, hard pimples, with little or no lymph, and never with any pus occurred in probably one case out of twenty or thirty. These spots, so unlike the small-pox, gave no trouble, and were of such short duration, that when I speak of eruptions I do not include them in the account; I include those only in which the eruptions resembled the small-pox: nor do I reckon among the eruptive cases, those in which, in a few instances, a rash broke out about the 14th day after inoculation, and which was as troublesome as the **Urticaria**."[138]

These spots which Pearson and other early vaccinators, including Jenner, discounted as being of no significance, were, in fact, an ominous portent of what was to follow. Here is Pearson's account in the spring of 1800 of the origin of the vaccine which led to the Petworth outbreak of smallpox:

> "In the month of October last I inoculated a child, two years of age, with the vaccine . . . The . . . disease took

> place with the usual appearances in the inoculated part, and affected the whole constitution in the ordinary manner; but a few eruptions broke out on the second or third day, after a slight fever; they were, however, only the red large pimples aforementioned, and, of course, not at all like the small-pox. Mr. Keate carried matter from this child to Brighthelmstone, where Mr. Barrett inoculated two children, who took the disease, and from one of these Mr. Keate inoculated three children. They all had the usual fever about the eighth day, and all had a number of eruptions except one, who had only five or six . . . Matter from these patients was sent to Petworth, where Mr. Andre informs me, he inoculated with it fourteen children. They all took the disease, and had eruptions like the variolous."[139]

This experience led Pearson to conclude that "from the occurrence of such [eruptive] cases in the practice of other inoculators in the last autumn and this winter, I now think it very unreasonable to doubt any longer, that . . . the genuine vaccine poison does occasionally produce a certain variety of the cow-pock, characterised by the appearance of pustules like those of the variola."[140] He added, however, that if the precaution of avoiding inoculation with matter from eruptive was observed, "not above one case with variolous-like eruptions will be produced among two hundred instances of inoculated cow-pock" and these eruptive cases were "not more severe than the ordinary kinds of inoculated small-pox."[141]

With further attenuation of the virus through arm-to-arm inoculation, however, Pearson came to modify this view (as did all his contemporaries), so that, by 1803, he was claiming that the vaccine then used, which was "principally, if not solely, that which has been generated successively in the human animal, beginning in the first instance with the matter of the London Cows,"[142] was a pure cowpox vaccine which had been contaminated "in a few cases" only with smallpox.[143] The capacity that the original vaccinators had for self-deception was almost limitless: as early as March, 1800, Pearson was claiming that "the character of the inoculated Cowpock are the same now, that they were in the first instance, directly from the animal"[144] — a claim which echoed an almost identical one made by Jenner about Woodville's vaccine at the end of 1799.[145] However, Pearson's much more extensive experience of this lymph — he was responsible for introducing it into the army and navy, as well as through his Vaccine Institution distributing it to virtually every country of the world[146] — meant that he was forced to acknowledge the continuation of eruptions. The report of the Vaccine-Pock Institution (which he was responsible for founding) for the years 1800, 1801 and 1802, mentioned the following kinds of eruption:

> "Where there was considerable fever, on the second or third day after this fever, in a very small proportion of cases, eruptions appeared, seldom exceeding twenty, which were either hard pimples, not unlike smallpox, but scarcely with any fluid in them . . . 2. In the summer season, especially in August, a rash often broke out on the tenth or eleventh day, alleviating the specific fever but exciting much general irritation. 3. Another kind of eruption, we were rather told of than saw, was small maculae, like the measles, or those of the scarlatina anginosa. 4. A common rash has appeared on the ninth day, with great inflammation of the inoculated part, and great discharge; and a second eruption, like millet seeds, without fever. 5. A kind of eruption now and then occurred in hot weather, five to ten days after the period of vaccine fever, which was a very irritating rash, of the urticaria kind . . ."[147]

This is a unique detailed description of the eruptions which sometimes accompanied vaccination at this time; the report claimed that in the majority of cases — 449 out of 500 — no such complications occurred[148] and it is clear that, from this evidence and that given by Woodville at about the same time and earlier discussed, the lymph had been attenuated very substantially to give mainly local symptoms characteristic of classical vaccination.

Abundant confirmation of the conclusions reached so far about Woodville's lymph is to be found through the study of contemporary medical journals. Moore, the first

Director of the National Vaccine Establishment, correctly stated in his *History of Vaccination* that "the medical journals at this time teemed with cases of pustular eruptions from vaccination."[149] Reports specifically mentioning pustular cases with lymph supplied by Woodville or Pearson in 1799 and 1800, came from Finmere near Buckingham,[150] Leeds,[151] Ketley in Shropshire,[152] Kings Lynn, Norfolk,[153] Leith in Scotland,[154] Cork in Ireland,[155] Hanover in Germany,[156] Paris,[157] and Rotterdam.[158] Additional references to pustular eruptions with vaccine used in Mortlake in Surrey,[159], Edinburgh,[160] Manchester,[161] Winslow, Bucks,[162] Chobham in Surrey,[163] Wolverhampton,[164] Montrose,[165] Lucca in Italy and the Cape of Good Hope,[166] appeared, but did not state the origin of the vaccine. We shall see later that there were similar reports from medical practitioners who used Jenner's stock. The accounts of the eruptions suggested that they varied from severe reactions in a majority of the cases, to light symptoms in only a small minority. In the first category was the report of T. M. Kelson of Sevenoaks, who wrote in May of 1800 of his experiences in the previous year:

> "Early in last Spring, Dr. Pearson . . . sent me some vaccine virus, with which I inoculated several persons; in two instances only it took effect; on a man and a little girl. The former about the ninth day became ill, and so continued for several days, when a few **pink, fiery-looking blisters** appeared on his body, and then followed a very numerous eruption, exactly like small-pox of the distinct kind; they took the usual course of variolous pustules, and the man did well. From one of those **pink vesications,** I inoculated his wife, and she had the **true cow-pox,** with only **local pustules** . . . From the woman I inoculated three children, and they all had eruptions of the **variolous kind,** and were very ill during the eruptive fever. From those I inoculated a few others, some of whom had eruptions, and some had not."[167]

A similar report was published by Dr. Redfearn of Kings Lynn: all three cases vaccinated with lymph sent by Pearson had pustules — the first had forty on the "face, hands and back", the second had an eruption "perfectly analogous to the variolous disease" which "appeared upon the face, neck, hands and legs, extending itself over the whole surface of the body", while the third only suffered from "a few eruptive spots" which "were observed upon the face and hands, not more in number than five or six."[168] The unambiguous nature of the inoculations were brought out in the descriptions of very severe reactions of the kind mentioned, for example, by Dr. John Walker of Leeds in an unpublished letter to Lettsom:

> "I was the first in this place to commence it [vaccination] but unfortunately Dr. Pearson sent me variolous matter instead of the vaccine, and I had a case or two of acute small pox, with a very copious eruption of Pustules . . . We even inoculated from one of these Patients, and the disease excited by it continued to present the variolous Symptoms, beyond the possibility of Doubt. These patients were not influenced by, or subjected to, the Small pox atmosphere. This threw a damp on the practice [in Leeds] for nearly twelve Months . . ."[169]

However, frequent and severe pustular eruptions were not characteristic of the majority of reports. More typical was the account by the Rev. Robert Holt of Finmere, who stated that of about three hundred inoculated with Woodville's lymph, only three had pustular eruptions — one with "a small pustule two inches from the incision", and the other two with "above one hundred pustules in different parts of their bodies, which assumed precisely the appearance of that given by inoculation, except that they were smaller."[170] The Rev. Holt sent some of this lymph to the Rev. W. Finch of St. Helens in November, 1799, and in his hands it produced even milder effects. Finch described a number of minor but very important symptoms which might have escaped a less scrupulous observer; he noted that in one child "a small red spot was discovered under its left thigh", another had "one pustule upon the nape of his neck" and "a few others had one or two red spots on different parts of their body, but none of them ever suppurated" — and this was out of a total of 714 cases.[171] The number of pustules that vaccinators observed partly depended on their definition of a pustule; as we have seen, both Woodville and Pearson claimed that by the year 1800, the number of pustules ranged from "not above one case . . . among two hundred" (Pearson) to "three or four cases out of one hundred" (Woodville). Most contemporaries seemed to have accepted that in order for an eruption to be characterised as pustular, it had to be associated with maturation and suppuration — otherwise the eruption was referred to as a spot or a pimple and not enumerated in the count of pustules. Also some practitioners had a similar experience to Woodville's, of a rapid decline in the number of pustules through arm-to-arm inoculation. The first reported vaccination at the Manchester Infirmary took place on the 16th April, 1799 and M. Ward, a resident surgeon, described the symptoms as follows:

> "The first patient . . had a confluent eruption; and . . . she was in so much danger, as to make me very anxious about her . . . a great number of pustules appeared on her neck, breast and arms; and . . . there is a plentiful crop on every part of her body."[172]

Other cases vaccinated at the same time also had pustules and later, at the end of 1800, W. Simmons summarised the history of vaccination in Manchester:

> "An eruption of pustules was, for some time, a pretty constant attendant on this inoculation; latterly, however, seldom any have appeared on distant parts of the body, and not more in number than three or four; the inflammation on the arm, together with pustular eruption on that part, and a slight febrile attack, have constituted all the signs of the disease."[173]

The increasingly localised nature of pustular eruptions (around the site of injection) was also Woodville's experience, and we will see this has some importance in explaining the nature of the changes to these inoculations of smallpox.

CHAPTER 5

Pustular Eruptions with Jenner's Stock of Vaccine

We have now reached the point in the book where we must consider Jenner's own experience of pustular eruptions with the vaccine he was using, as well as that of medical practitioners who were supplied by him. At the outset, it must be said that Jenner was not the most reliable witness as to the nature of his own vaccine; for example, in publishing a letter from Henry Cline on the use of his Berkeley lymph in the summer of 1798, he changed an original statement in the letter — "The ulcer was not large enough to contain a pea, therefore I have not converted it into an issue as I intended" — to — "There were no eruptions."[174] This deliberate distortion of the evidence might be justified on the grounds that Jenner was trying to bring out that his original lymph was not accompanied by pustular eruptions, but it does indicate that one must treat his claims and statements on this subject with some caution. Similarly, when he sent Ring a supply of Woodville's lymph in September, 1799, he claimed to "have seen no pustules produced by it . . . except in a single instance, (and) they did not maturate."[175] — and yet as we have seen, he admitted to Lord Egremont that he had seen pustules on his "first patients" with this vaccine.

The first general reference to eruptions occurred in a letter from Jenner to De Carro on the 27th November, 1799:

> "When the **Areola** has spread wide around the inoculated Pustule I have sometimes seen a rash upon the Patient, and sometimes several pimples, small, hard and of a reddish colour have shown themselves on different parts of the body, some of which have contained a perceptible fluid at their apex. But this appearance is very rare . . ."[176]

In the same letter, Jenner claimed that with Woodville's lymph, "The Pustules, as the disease made its progress from one patient to another soon began to decrease in number, and now they are become quite extinct, the matter producing appearances exactly similar to that newly taken from the Pock on the Nipple of the Cow."[177] As Woodville himself described a small proportion of his cases still experiencing pustules at this time, it would appear that Jenner had reached this conclusion from his own experience of declining pustules, rather than from Woodville's published accounts.

As we have seen, in his letter to Lord Egremont in December, 1799, Jenner referred to using Woodville's lymph, seeing "a few pustules" on his "first patients" — but in his "subsequent inoculations there were none". In the same letter, he claimed to have "sometimes seen, perhaps in one case in a hundred, a few scattered pimples about the body, and sometimes rashes . . .".[178] The ambiguity of language employed by Jenner — first describing the eruptions as pustules, then referring to them as pimples — characterised his later statements on the subject. In his pamphlet written at the end of 1799, he stated that he had been supplied with some of Woodville's lymph, and that "In the first instance it produced a few pustules which did not maturate; but in subsequent cases none appeared."[179] Similarly he noted that some of his correspondents had "mentioned the appearance of Small Pox-like eruptions at the commencement of their inoculations" — but he qualified this by pointing out that "the matter was derived from the original stock at the Small Pox Hospital"[180] although from descriptions and quotes from his correspondents' letters, it would appear that he had himself been supplying them with this stock of Woodville's lymph. Yet within a month or so he was denying that he had ever experienced pustules, like those characteristic of smallpox:

> ". . . from the commencement of my inoculation with the vaccine virus to the present day, no pustules, similar to the variolous, have in any one instance appeared. I have seen rashes, and sometimes (though very rarely) I have observed a few scattered pimples about the body . . ."[181]

Five months later, he repeated this statement, with a minor qualification about pustules appearing in two cases: "I have seen pimples excited by the cow-pox, with sometimes a little fluid at their apex; and, in two instances, a vaccine pustule, resembling that on the arm produced by inoculation; but in no instance, a small-pox-like pustule."[182]

In a letter to Waterhouse, dated the 4th March, 1801, Jenner came nearest to making an admission that eruptions were fairly common accompaniments to vaccination:

> "It is by no means uncommon to see an appearance something like tooth rash. I have seen too, though very rarely, the vaccine pustule, once upon the chin of an adult, and in two or three instances among children. But every thing of the eruptive kind I have ever seen has been too immaterial to merit notice . . ."[183]

His last statement made on the subject was to the Royal College of Physicians Vaccination Committee on the 19th February, 1807; when asked whether eruptions formed a part of the disease of vaccination, his answer was recorded as follows:

> "They do, but they are rare. They consist in minute Vesicles thinly scattered, and contain a limpid fluid in their Apex, and bear no resemblance to the Pustules of Small Pox. He has not seen more than seven such Cases, nor has he generally looked for them because he considers them insignificant. In three or four Instances, he has seen Urticaria."[184]

The tone of this statement — "nor has he generally looked for them" — reveals a defensive mentality, which perhaps conceals facts too awkward and inconvenient to be accepted and therefore observed in an impartial manner. This is certainly suggested by the evidence of other practitioners using Jenner's vaccine, but it is only possible to conclude that from Jenner's own general statements, the case about small-pox pustular eruptions is not definitely proved one way or the other.

The first person to use Jenner's stock of vaccine on any scale was Dr. Joseph Marshall of Eastington in Gloucestershire. He wrote two letters to Jenner — one in April and the other in September, 1799 — which were both published. In the first, he described how he had inoculated 107 people with Woodville's lymph, and claimed that "in only one or two of the cases have any eruptions appeared than those around the spot where the matter was inserted, and those near the infected parts."[185] It is not clear what the nature of the eruptions around the site of injection was — this kind of sattelite eruption was thought of by Ring as characteristic of inoculated smallpox. The "one or two" cases of other pustular eruption are not at all precisely described, although in his second letter, he did indicate that he was using the term pustule to refer to an eruption which had maturated.[186] Marshall further claimed that there was no substantial difference between the Woodville and Kentish Town Farm lymph that Jenner had sent him, but he did not discuss this in any detail. This is not inconsistent with the accounts of other practitioners who had used Woodville's lymph; we have seen, Pearson claimed that "variolous-like eruptions" only occurred in about one in two hundred cases. What emerged as a critical point from our review of the literature was the existence of other kinds of eruptions, not typical of classical smallpox, but modified through arm-to-arm inoculation to such an extent as to appear like an eruption of spots rather than orthodox smallpox pustules. Woodville, Pearson and Jenner tended to discount these "pimples" in their general accounts of the results of their inoculations; it is possible that Marshall treated them in the same way.

The critical importance of the definition of a pustule emerged in the next published account of the independent use of Jenner's vaccine. Dr. J. Evans of Ketley in Shropshire included pustules which did not maturate in his account of the eruptions which followed vaccination — of sixty-eight patients, "thirty-nine had an **eruption,** but only two . . . (had) pustules (which) arrived to a state of maturation, and those imperfectly."[187] Evans published a detailed account of the effects of vaccination, with the additional interest of a comparison of the results of using lymph derived from Pearson as against that coming directly from Jenner. He wrote two letters to Woodville in September, 1799, of which the following is an extract:

". . . I was particularly careful in the choice of a lancet that had never been used for any other purpose . . . I began to inoculate on the 11th May, and continued the practice till the end of June. The [first] vaccine virus which I [used] . . . was originally sent . . . by Dr. Pearson of St. George's Hospital. On the 8th of June I used that sent me by Dr. Jenner, and no other during the remainder of my practice. The appearance of an eruption on the first two patients surprised me greatly, as well as those subsequently inoculated, till I read your "Reports", when my mind was relieved; and after I was favoured with vaccine virus by Dr. Jenner, I was convinced, from the exact similarity of its effects, that . . . [the first] was genuine."[188]

Although Evans described a case with "many distinct pustules on different parts" of the body, and stated that the parents of the patients were "so well satisfied" with the results of the inoculation "from its similarity to the smallpox", he admitted that in "the vaccine patients . . . their indisposition in general [was] less severe."[189] An important difference was in the distribution and nature of the pustules:

> "The greatest number of pustules was generally around the part where the matter was inserted; they had the appearance that the small-pox has during the eruptive fever, and all (except what I have before mentioned) went off without arriving to a state of maturation."[190]

At the end of his second letter, Evans listed each case inoculated and the number of pustules which resulted. He unfortunately does not date the cases or indicate which were vaccinated with the lymph sent by Pearson as against that sent by Jenner. He mentioned that he had used Pearson's lymph for about four weeks, and Jenner's for just over three weeks; if we divide his sample into two (he listed his cases consecutively in the order that they were inoculated), this will give us some quantitative comparison between the two lymphs. Of the first 34 cases, 23 had pustules totalling 442 (an average of 19 pustules); of the second 34, 16 had pustules totalling 392 (an average over 24 pustules). This evidence would be more or less conclusive proof that Jenner's stock of vaccine at this time was derived from Woodville's attenuated smallpox strain, except for one possible complication of interpretation. As well as vaccinating children with the Pearson and Jenner lymphs, Evans inoculated other members of the same family wherever he could with smallpox virus. He did this so as to be able to compare the results of the two forms of inoculation, but it obviously complicates the situation by raising the possibility that some of those vaccinated were infected by the smallpox virus of their siblings. In practice, this does not appear to have happened because Evans tells us that the:

> "vaccine Patients were sooner affected . . . and the disease [was] of much shorter duration than those inoculated with variolous virus . . . Several of the [vaccine] patients slept with others who had full crops of small-pox pustules, without being in the least degree affected."[191]

This is consistent with what we know of the shorter incubation period for more attenuated forms of a disease like smallpox, and Evans unambiguously indicates that there was no secondary infection from contact with smallpox virus. Without details of the timing of symptom development, however, and in the light of the fact of contact with inoculated smallpox cases, we must conclude that there is an element of doubt on Evans's evidence about the identical nature of Pearson's and Jenner's vaccines.

The next independent evidence on Jenner's vaccine comes from an article probably written in the autumn of 1799 by Pearson, but published in the following year. He quoted two examples of Jenner's lymph producing pustules:

> "1. In a person inoculated by Dr. Jenner, in the country, who came to town, and was under the care of Mr. Cotton, 'the eruptions bore much resemblance to the inoculated Small-pox, in number from twelve to twenty'. See Mr. Cotton's letter to Dr. Pearson. 2. . . . 'I have', says Mr. Ring, in his letter to Dr. Pearson, 'inoculated thirty patients with matter given to me by Mr. Paytherus, and to him by Dr. Jenner. One of these had about 150 pustules; these were not distinguishable from variolous ones by any diagnostics with which I am acquainted. The

matter was purulent; became perfectly opaque, and on exsication, formed a scab as large as that left by the Small-pox."[192]

As Jenner never repudiated either of these two statements, we must assume that they refer to incidents which occurred as described. There is no further reference in the literature to Mr. Cotton's patient, and as far as I am aware, the letter quoted by Pearson has never been published in full. The second incident involving Ring's patients was, however, further discussed by Ring; in a letter written on the 6th May, 1800, he stated that "in the first five cases [of inoculation with Jenner's vaccine and supplied by Mr. Paytherus], one was attended with a pustular eruption."[193] He later argued that although these "varioliform pustules could not be accounted for . . . the variolous miasmata are invisible agents; and almost continually float in the atmosphere of London."[194] It is of course possible that an isolated outbreak of smallpox inflection of unknown origin could have occurred, but this explanation becomes much less plausible in the light of a more general remark made by Ring (on the 6th May, 1800) on the subject of eruptions:

". . . I have seen a number of persons inoculated with supposed vaccine matter, who had eruptions in a trifling degree, both in my own practice and in that of others; but the eruptions in general were not pustulous. They rather resembled the tooth-rash than the small-pox; and were neither attended with danger nor inconvenience. In some instances a small vesicle has appeared, not altogether unlike that on the arm; but without any material inflammation."[195]

The language of this statement is virtually identical to that of Pearson in his accounts of "non-variolous" eruptions of spots and pimples; and although they appeared to Ring to be "neither attended with danger nor inconvenience", like Pearson's lymph, the vaccine which produced them was later to produce full-blown cases of smallpox which probably created a minor epidemic. Ring's admission that eruptions did occur with the lymph that he was using is important, because, as we have seen, he and Jenner after the autumn of 1799, began to use a common stock of vaccine which was used interchangeably.

One piece of evidence that goes against the line of argument being developed in this book must now be considered. On the 24th March, 1800, Stromeyer wrote a letter giving an account of his experience of vaccination in Hanover in Germany:

> "This year we have inoculated forty persons, as well with the vaccine matter received of Dr. Pearson, as that of Dr. Jenner, all of which went properly through the disease. Betwixt the London and Gloucester vaccine matter, it appears to me, there subsists an essential difference. The London matter produces frequently an eruption of small pimples, but they disappear within a day or two at the furthest. Dr. Pearson calls these eruptions pimples. The Gloucester matter has never produced this effect here; but it frequently **occasioned ulcerations of the inoculated part, of a tedious and long duration, which the former matter never did;** on account of which I now only make use of Dr. Pearson's vaccine matter."[196]

This is strong evidence for a difference in the nature of Jenner's and Pearson's lymph, and from the descriptions given by Stromeyer, the former had all the classical characteristics of a genuine cowpox vaccine, whereas the latter gave rise to symptoms more typical of an attenuated smallpox lymph. However, there are two important points to be made about this conclusion. Firstly, it should be noted that Stromeyer rejected Jenner's lymph in favour of that from Pearson, on account of the severe ulceration of the vaccine tumour. This ironically, was one of the reasons for Jenner's preference for Woodville's lymph over those he had previously used, and it is likely to be a part of the explanation as to why he continued to use the Woodville strain as the basis of his main stock, in spite of the availability of other strains of vaccine directly derived from cowpox. The second point concerns the timing of Stromeyer's report; he had been using both the Pearson and Jenner lymphs for the first two or three months of 1800, and we know that Jenner had used the Kentish Town cowpox vaccine at the end of 1799, and had "dispersed it among others" at about that time. In the pamphlet written by him giving his information, he indicated that he had used the Kentish Town lymph on an experimental basis, and was going to continue to use the Woodville lymph as his main stock. It is likely that the vaccine that he had sent to Stromeyer (at the end of 1799 or beginning of 1800?) was the Kentish Town stock, but that future supplies sent out by him were the Woodville lymph. The origin of the vaccine that Stromeyer obtained from Jenner is entirely hypothetical, but the above conclusion is consistent with the weight of evidence both already and about to be considered. It is also important to note, that no other account pointing to a difference between the Woodville/Pearson and Jenner lymphs has come to light — and given what we know about the characteristics of the two types of vaccine, we would expect if Jenner had widely used the Kentish Town lymph or any other vaccine directly derived from cowpox, this to have shown up in the abundant literature on the subject at this time.

On the 24th April, 1800, T. S. Gooch Esq. of Hadleigh, Suffolk, wrote to Jenner giving an account of the vaccination of 611 people with lymph sent originally by Jenner:

> "I see by your last publication you suppose it impossible for a person inoculated with the pure **uncontaminated** cowpox virus to have pustules; I beg leave to mention on that subject that we have had six people with evident pustules, from which we might have inoculated. Two of them had pustules on the eye, and four on the inoculated arm near the elbow . . . We had our virus from Mrs. Gooch's sister, Lady Rouse, who had it immediately from you."[197]

A similar proportion of a small number of pustular eruptions was experienced by Dr. R. J. Thornton, who obtained a supply of Jenner's vaccine from Ring. Initially he inoculated eight cases on October the 4th, of which only one had a "solitary pustule near the inoculated one"; of 23 later cases which were described, one had "an attempt towards forming a kind of eruption, one pustule appearing on the breast, and another on the cheek . . ."[198] Thornton sent a supply of this vaccine to William Harrison of Ulverstone, who reported on the 1st December, 1800, that out of twenty to thirty cases inoculated, one "had three pustules on her face."[199] The number of eruptions of "pimples" and more ambiguous forms of pustules is unknown, the writers of these reports typically not discussing questions of definition. In the following year, J. Blount of Birmingham wrote to Jenner (on the 14th June, 1801) to describe the results of using a supply of the former's vaccine; of three cases discussed, two did not take,

> "and the third was taken to a distance by the mother the day after inoculation, so that I never saw the child after; but I have since heard, that the mother returned in a few days with the child, who had about fifty eruptions, of what she thought was the **Small-pox.** The disease appearing so slight, she did not think it necessary to trouble me with it . . ."[200]

It must have been common for both medical practitioners and the parents of patients, to make light of the small proportion of minor pustular eruptions that did occur with vaccination in this early period. But there is some evidence now to be considered, that taking vaccine from such an eruptive pustule could lead in some instances to a restoration of the virulence of the attenuated smallpox virus used.

It was from such a pustule that one of the most active supporters of vaccination propagated a species of vaccine which degenerated into a severe form of smallpox almost identical to that experienced at Petworth. I refer to the experience of Benjamin Waterhouse, known as the "American Jenner" because of his role in introducing vaccination into the United States. I will discuss Waterhouse's experience in some detail, because it illustrates better than any of the other examples, the variolous nature of Jenner's main stock of vaccine.

CHAPTER 6

Waterhouse's Use of Jenner's Vaccine in the United States and the Marblehead Smallpox Epidemic

At the beginning of July, 1800, Waterhouse received vaccine from Haygarth of Bath, which had been "procured from Dr. Jenner's stock by Mr. Creaser."[201] On the 8th July, he commenced his practice by inoculating seven of his family;[202] unfortunately he did not give detailed descriptions of the results of these early vaccinations but enough emerges from the literature to indicate the nature of the virus involved. The first person inoculated was one of his sons, resulting in a purely local reaction, with "no pustules on his body". From the latter's arm, Waterhouse took lymph and vaccinated a second son, three years of age — with the result of "a full maturated pustule, four inches from the place of inoculation."[203] With matter from this pustule, an infant sister and a nursemaid were vaccinated:

> "They both went through the disease with . . . symptoms . . . very similar to those of the lighter kind from inoculation for the smallpox, viz. a slight dizziness and nausea, watery eyes, chilliness, soreness of the flesh, usually called by the common people in this country, "bones-ache", a general lassitude, transient pains in the stomach, loins and head, with a disinclination to animal food and exercise . . . The striking similarity of symptoms has induced some practitioners in this country . . . to conclude, that the **kine-pox** (cow-pox) was only a variety of the smallpox."[204]

Waterhouse did not give a detailed description of the number of pustules involved in these early cases, and this was partly a function of his confusion about the correct nature of vaccination. He had taken material from a pustule other than at the site of injection, and clearly believed that eruptions were a normal part of the disease, concluding that the vaccinations of six of his family had proceeded "exactly as described by Woodville and Jenner."[205] In a letter to Ring, Waterhouse, after describing the fully maturated pustule four inches away from the site of injection in his second child, admitted "numbers, besides his own patients, who have had a considerable crop of pustules."[206] These pustules could not be accounted for by secondary smallpox infection, for as Ring pointed out, there was no evidence of smallpox in the area when Waterhouse commenced his vaccinations.[207]

As a result of his experience, Waterhouse found himself initially in agreement with Woodville and Pearson:

> "Dr. W. and Dr. P. contended that the vaccine matter was capable of producing small-pox pustules with all their phenomena as to contagion, etc. and that the vaccine disease was attended like the small-pox with pustules all over the body. This error is conspicuous in my first publication."[208]

By the middle of November, 1800, Waterhouse began to claim (like Woodville, Jenner and Pearson) that the effects of vaccination became attenuated by arm-to-arm inoculation. Other evidence on the results of vaccination in October, 1800, seem to confirm this conclusion. In a private letter to Dr. Lyman Spalding whom he had supplied with a stock of vaccine, Waterhouse warned on the 12th October "that you must take the matter from the inoculated part . . . and never from the pustules that rarely occur"[209] (presumably by this time he had become aware of what the symptoms of vaccination should consist of). Three days previously, Spalding had written to another medical colleague, stating that of fifteen people vaccinated with the lymph supplied by Waterhouse, "one only, has the appearance of eruption."[210] In October, 1800, an anonymous author stated that "in eight instances out of ten, the whole visible effect of the inoculated Kine-Pox is confined to the neighbourhood of the incision . . ."[211] It therefore appears that by early October, pustular cases were occurring, but rather infrequently. But during the month of October, very disturbing reports began to reach Waterhouse of epidemics of smallpox in Marblehead and Beverley, near Boston, which were reputed to have been started by vaccination. Waterhouse, frightened that this would discredit both the new practice and himself, explained at some length his own role in the affair, in a letter written on the 14th November and published in the local newspaper:

> "A report having prevailed for several days past that the kine-pox had appeared in Marblehead with symptoms of unheard of virulency and even **contagion,** I feel myself particularly bound to give the public an history of the facts which gave rise to it . . . On the 14th October, Dr. Elisha Story of Marblehead, sent to me for the kine-pox matter, which I immediately sent him. His son, who did the message, informed me that his father had imported some from London, and had inoculated his sister with it, but having waited **twelve days,** and finding no symptoms to follow, considered the matter was bad, and therefore wished some of mine. Three days after, viz. on the 17th, Dr. Story wrote to me, that he had not used the matter I sent, for his daughter had that morning broken out with the disease, which was **fifteen days** after he had inoculated her. Even at the time I was struck with the description of it. He described the symptoms as very high, 'accompanied with a great number of pustules, **small and hard in the flesh, with a small margin of inflammation** around the same.' Appearances that never occur in the Kine-Pox. About this time I inoculated the son of Dr. Drury (the other Physician of Marblehead) for the Kine-Pox, and thereby allowed his father a crop of matter for his own practice. When I heard that the Kine-Pox was raging at Marblehead and Beverley, and that some were blind with it, and that moreover proved contagious; and when I recollected the symptoms, as described by Dr. Story, my mind was strongly impressed that it was not the Kine-Pox, nor a mixture of it but the **Small-Pox.** On the 12th of the present month [November], Mr. **Josiah Story** called upon me again, saying that his father wished for some of my Kine-Pox matter, for that the Kine Pox, **or something like it,** had arisen from the matter which he had imported, but with very alarming appearances . . . But what riveted my opinion that it was the Small-Pox, was his saying **'that the matter which his father inoculated,**

was taken from the arm of a sailor, on the passage between London and Marblehead,' by one of his brothers who was on board the ship; which sailor was probably inoculated with Small Pox before he left England; or else was inoculated with the Kine-Pox, and previously caught the Small Pox . . . As to the opinion that the kine-pox will increase in virulency until it finally becomes the small-pox, I never heard nor experienced any thing that favours the notion, but quite the reverse. If we are to judge the force of the disease by the number of pustules, it certainly becomes milder as it recedes from the cow. It is well known that cold diminishes the activity of febrile poisons . . . I have never seen a case of the kine-pox any how alarming . . ."[212]

This version of the epidemic at Marblehead has never been questioned by medical historians, and this is largely because nearly all the information published about it came from Waterhouse, and he both suppressed and distorted crucial facts which were deeply embarrassing to himself and his practice of vaccination. The reader will note from the above account that there were **"no symptoms"** by twelve days in Dr. Story's daughter; if Waterhouse were correct in believing that she had inadvertently been inoculated with smallpox, she would almost certainly have had a strong local reaction well within this period. Smallpox having broken out in her on the fifteenth day without previous symptoms, she is likely to have been infected with natural smallpox (i.e. through respiratory infection). Waterhouse categorically denied that any of his own vaccinated cases had the kind of severe symptoms that could have been the source of contagion, and in his letter he admits only to vaccinating Dr. Drury's son about the same time as the infection of Dr. Story's daughter. Both these statements can be shown to be false — and they can be shown to be false by statements later made by Waterhouse himself.

On the 15th December, an anonymous author under the title of "Anti-Synopsis" wrote a letter to a local newspaper complaining about the failure of vaccination to protect against smallpox: "of 50 persons there [Marblehead] inoculated with the kine-pox matter, procured from the most approved sources, and regularly exhibiting all the symptoms of the disease with inflammation, pustules, etc., only about one tenth were protected from the ravages of the small-pox . . ."[213] The confusion in this contemporary account is apparent: the author clearly believed that "kine-pox inoculation" was a pustular disease, but appears not to have realised that much of the smallpox amongst the vaccinated cases was probably due to the inoculation of smallpox virus. Waterhouse was concerned to defend vaccination against the charge that it failed to protect against smallpox, as well as defend his own reputation (presumably he was the "most approved sources" referred to). On the 20th December, he wrote defending vaccination and elaborating his own role in the Marblehead epidemic:

> ". . . I inoculated two, and but two inhabitants of Marblehead. One was a person whose name I have forgotten, who said he would return to me in six days, that I might see if his inoculation had **taken**. But he returned no more. As I never saw him under the disorder, I cannot be answerable for him. The other man was the son of a practitioner [Dr. Drury], a boy of about eight or nine years of age. His father brought him to my house in Cambridge. I put the thread in his arm, and gave his father a small portion of the same, but never saw nor heard any more of the boy afterwards, and of course I never knew whether he ever had the genuine **local infection,** and **specific fever,** which constitutes that pecular distemper, which I have said and still believe secures the human system from the small-pox. Yet from this boy's arm, was taken, as I am informed, all the matter, with which all the others in Marblehead were inoculated. If the matter therefore, which I used, did not give the genuine disease in the **first** instance, which happens very frequently, then all the cases that followed it must of course be **spurious,** and absolutely incapable of securing the system from an attack of small-pox . . . For about two or three weeks in the month of November the matter seemed to have undergone **a deterioration** in my hands. I inoculated several

persons four or five times over before I could communicate the disease. To three of four I never could communicate it . . . I have entertained an opinion . . . that **the kine pox matter becomes milder as it recedes from the Cow,** and that in process of time it gets worn out . . . When it is known that all the vaccine matter hitherto used in America (some received at Ipswich excepted) came from **less than two inches** of infected thread which I received from Bath, in England last June, this idea will not appear altogether absurd . . ."[214]

Waterhouse conceded that vaccination had failed to protect against smallpox but continued to argue that his own cases had nothing to do with the beginning of the epidemic as such. He was prepared to admit that the vaccine had deteriorated even in his own practice, although characteristically he implied that it was the incompetence of someone else (Dr. Drury) which had given rise to the "spurious" cases in Marblehead (two years later Waterhouse made this implicit charge explicit by accusing Drury of not following his "directions respecting the **time** of taking the matter."[215]) In this letter of the 20th December there are no details of the timing of Waterhouse's vaccination of the two Marblehead cases, and no description of their symptoms — in spite of being given "a plain and candid history" of the whole sequence of events by Drs. Story, Drury and others, in visits to Salem and Marblehead before Waterhouse's first letter of the 14th November.[216]

Two years after these events of 1800, Waterhouse published a further description of what had happened which totally contradicted his initial account. He reiterated his view of the origin of the Marblehead epidemic — the unintended inoculation of smallpox virus by Dr. Story with matter taken from the sailor's arm — but gave details of his own practice of vaccination and of the cases that he had inoculated in Marblehead, which brings into question the conventional medical historical view of these events. The first major contradiction of his earlier evidence came in a statement about his first letter to the local newspapers:

"I felt it my duty in November of the same year [1800] to acquaint the public, through the medium of the news-

> paper, that the kinepock had, in many places, degenerated from its original mild character, and that this deviation appeared from the inoculator taking his matter from the pustule at **too late a period**."[217]

The reader will note by comparing this with the quote from the published November letter that Waterhouse turned the latter upside down; whereas in the published letter he claimed that the "kine-pock" was becoming milder through arm-to-arm inoculation, two years later in 1802 he was admitting that it had become severer. The reference to taking matter at too late a period originated from an idea of Jenner's, that most spurious cases were due to the timing of taking the vaccine.[218] No mention is to be found in any of Waterhouse's newspaper letter or other writings for the year of 1800 of a warning to the public about severer cases, but on the contrary the reverse is true: he publicly denied stories that the vaccine matter had deteriorated into smallpox, and stated that the lymph had become milder to the point of becoming "worn out". Yet his 1802 publication gives the details of a vaccine that had become highly virulent to the point of becoming very dangerous to those infected with it; immediately after given an account of the Marblehead epidemic, Waterhouse confessed:

> "I wish not to conceal from the public, that about the latter end of the autumn, or beginning of the winter of 1801, I perceived that the vaccine disease had deviated from its original character, and assumed a face with which I was not acquainted. I endeavoured to account for this change of countenance by persuading myself that the virus became milder as it receded from the cow; and that it would at length become effete by passing through a given number of human subjects . . . But this notion was encumbered with several difficulties, as many cases arose in direct opposition to it; for instead of becoming milder, they were in fact severer in all their symptoms. This induced some to adopt a notion directly opposite; that the small-pox was at its origin the cow-pox . . . for when the small-pox appeared first at Marblehead, it was very

universally believed that it was the cow, or kine-pock, verging in malignity to the small-pox . . . I silently entertained another whim, that the cold weather aggravated this disease . . ."[219]

He had not only persuaded himself that the virus became milder with use, but had written two long newspaper letters attempting to convince the public at large of the same notion. In his 1802 publication, he came near also to admitting that the people of Marblehead had been right about the origin of smallpox in their town:

> "All those cases, where there were violent inflammation, deap seated ulceration, eruptions, and heavy febrile symptoms, were not the true kine-pock, but a malady generated by a highly acrid, putrid matter; or in one word, poisonous matter, taken from under a scab, or from an open ulcer, long after the specific virus was annihilated. I used in three or four persons some shining, glazy looking thread, which was dispensed in great profusion in Boston and its neighbourhood, in the autumn of 1800, and it produced in every case very distressing, if not alarming symptoms; severer in most respects, than the ordinary ones in the variolous inoculation . . . I am still ignorant of the genealogy of this matter; I only know that it was not the vaccine virus, whatever might have been its origin . . . I had but few cases of this cast, but nevertheless heard loud complaints from others . . . Had these severe cases continued, I should have relinquished the practice, and advised everybody else to do likewise."[220]

In fact, Waterhouse did relinquish the practice at this time, and only recommenced it with a further supply of vaccine from Jenner in 1801. The "shining, glazy looking thread" was reminiscent of the "shining, smooth, black" scabs that Pearson had experienced with the use of Woodville's lymph — and given the common origin of Waterhouse's vaccine (Jenner's stock, originating in the arm of Ann Bumpus) and Pearson's, it is likely that they were both experiencing a similar resurgence of virulence in the attenuated smallpox virus that they were using.

Marblehead, being in the neighbourhood of Boston (Waterhouse described it as "a considerable sea-port 16 miles from Boston")[221] was presumably one of the areas in which this virulent species of vaccine was used. Waterhouse never explicitly accepted responsibility for the epidemic, although he admitted that "purulent matter . . . always fails in communicating the genuine kine pox. The matter, used at Marblehead, was purulent . . ."[222] and he himself drew a parallel between the Marblehead experience and that at Petworth and elsewhere:

> "The like occurrences took place at Geneva, and at several places in England, especially at Petworth, where the virus . . . gave a **spurious** [disease] . . . the effects formed a counterpart to the disasters at Marblehead."[223]

The "purulent matter" used at Marblehead was presumably that used by Waterhouse on the two cases inoculated by him. He gives further details of these in his later publication, which reveal even more contradictions of his initial accounts. Most importantly, the identity of the first Marblehead person to be vaccinated by Waterhouse is revealed: this "was a young gentleman, Mr. F., a particular connection of Dr. S. [Story] . . . [he] was an assistant inoculator, and in some instances nurse, during the whole time that disorder [smallpox] was passing through the town . . ."[224] This implies that he was vaccinated before the beginning of the epidemic — which would make it very likely (given what we know about the virulent nature of Waterhouse's vaccine) that he was the source of the epidemic, which was reputed to have started with Dr. Story's daughter. It is possible that Mr. F. was vaccinated by Waterhouse on the 14th October, and was the carrier of the virus that the latter had arranged to send to Story during the middle of October. That at least one of the two cases had been vaccinated before the beginning of the epidemic is tacitly admitted by Waterhouse in the statement that "previously to this sad accident [the spreading of smallpox through Marblehead], Dr. Drury had inoculated about forty persons, from the arm of his own son whom I had vaccinated . . ."[225]

Dr. Story did give some account — although unfortunately with little detail of timing and symptomology — which enables us to understand the origins of the Marblehead epidemic a bit further. On the 4th May, 1801, he wrote to the Massachusetts Medical Society, describing what he knew about the new "kine-pox inoculation":

> ". . . Early in October last my son brot me home from London some Kinepox matter as the Physician who inoculated 4 Men on board his ship informed him, of which matter I inoculated eight of my family, only one took, & broke out the 17 day and contrary to my expectation produced that fatal disease the Small pox; however, in the first instances it appeared very mild, and it was the opinion of the Medical Gentlemen who saw the Patients at that time, that it was an intermediate disease, between the kine and small pox, at least, that was their opinion then. I have never had an opportunity of inoculating for the Kine pox — therefore can say little about it. A Mr. Willm Fittyplace who was inoculated by Dr. Waterhouse for the Kine pox, was conversant with the Small pox in the natural way & by inoculation, being an assistant inoculator under me during the Small pox last fall . . ."[226]

This letter confirms that Story inoculated his daughter with matter taken from a sailor's arm, but it gives the additional information that in seven other members of his family it gave no reaction whatsoever, and that it did not break out in his daughter until the seventeenth day (it is not clear whether this was after the date of inoculation, or the day in the month). Without additional evidence about the timing of symptoms and the exposure of this daughter to other possible sources of smallpox virus, it is impossible to be sure how she contracted the disease. Story does reveal the name of Waterhouse's patient Mr. F — Mr. Fittyplace — and as the latter was Story's assistant (helping in the mass variolation which followed the outbreak of smallpox), it is certain that he would have been in contact with the Story family during the period of initial infection. It is not possible to say from the existing evidence whether Story's daughter caught smallpox from Fittyplace or not, but the fact that none of the other Story children were affected by their ostensible cowpox inoculation, and that the daughter was not affected until the fifteenth (seventeenth?) day, even at the site of injection, makes it likely that she caught smallpox from Fittyplace, who in turn had been infected by Waterhouse through his contaminated inoculations. We do not know for sure that Fittyplace did get smallpox from Waterhouse, but Story's reference to the patients in the plural getting a smallpox-like disease from the ostensible kine-pox inoculations, would suggest this. It is also important to note that Story conducted no further vaccinations and that the forty or so conducted in Marblehead were carried out by Drury.

Sixty-eight people died from smallpox in Marblehead.[227] There were no other epidemic outbreaks but there were threatened epidemics. For example, at the end of October, 1800, the Rev. William Bentley of Salem, visited the neighbouring town of Beverley to witness the results of introducing the new practice of vaccination:

> "October 30 . . . Went to Beverley to see the first example of the Kine Pox in our neighbourhood. Dr. Whitney inoculated his own four children, the three eldest females. The symptoms were long and severe, with shivering, pain and fainting, and lasted six days. The eldest had few pustules, but very sore, was of a slender habit. The second daughter had it less severe in the symptoms but more pustules and very sore. The third daughter of more full habit had the symptoms very severely and was loaded especially about the face, arms and feet. The Son was very faint, and feeble, has few pustules, but great debility, just recovering. As I found the pustules, they were large and the pustulous matter more clear than commonly in the smallpox, but not essentially different. The pustules did pit, were not much inflamed at the edges, were confluent, and of bright yellow when drying away."[228]

Not surprisingly, the Whitney family became "firmly persuaded that it was the smallpox" that they were suffering from. Bentley did not explicitly state the source of the vaccine used, but given that nearly all the lymph used in America came from Waterhouse at this time, and that he admitted sending out such virulent vaccine to the neighbourhood of Boston, it is likely that Dr. Whitney had obtained it from him. Bentley at the end of November did specifically link the severe cases with Waterhouse, and unambiguously labelled them as smallpox: "we hear that Waterhouse has written to some patients his apprehensions of some of his variolous matter."[229] Bentley goes on to describe how Dr. Little of Salem inoculated his own child and others with "kine pox", and implies that the results were similar to those at Beverley, for "Dr. Little by sending the patients inoculated in his own home, to the hospital upon the first alarm has prevented much public uneasiness, and no one yet had the Natural small pox in Salem."[230] Town Meetings were called at both Beverley and Salem to consider action to contain a possible smallpox epidemic, but although wide discretionary powers were given to the Selectmen and Health Committee, the prohibition of all further forms of inoculations appears to have been sufficient. Bentley mentioned on the 11th November that "in consequence of the imprudent management of the Cow Pox, the real Small Pox has been spread over Marblehead", and added that "there are reports that the Physician who incautiously spread the disease has been shot at with a pistol."[231] Waterhouse did not escape his share of the blame; writing in 1806 of a visit to Marblehead some years previously, he stated that "I . . . did not feel disposed to proceed **alone** to **Marblehead,** as I had heard the common people were highly exasperated, and had uttered threatening speeches against me, whom they considered as the first cause of their great calamity."[232] He eventually persuaded them of his innocence by vaccinating his coach driver with lymph received in the spring of 1801, and demonstrating the "true" character of the "kine-pox" — "They all pronounced it different from any inoculation they ever saw . . ."[233] (That this was proof of the contaminated nature of his own earlier vaccination including those in Marblehead, seems to have escaped Waterhouse.)

As a result of his experiences with this strain of vaccine, Waterhouse wrote to Jenner for a fresh supply. Ring described Waterhouse's approach to Jenner and what ensued:

> "Dr. Waterhouse . . . sent to Dr. Jenner for a fresh supply of matter; and requested that he might have some that was as recent from the cow as possible. That it was not practicable, or necessary to procure; since it was well known to Dr. Jenner . . . that the matter suffers no degeneracy, by repeated inoculation, in the human frame. The first supply which proved successful in the hands of Dr. Waterhouse . . . was . . . from the stock of Dr. Jenner. Dr. Waterhouse is again supplied from the same stock, with matter which has not suffered the least diminution of its original virtue."[234]

Jenner himself wrote a long letter on the 4th March, 1801, to Waterhouse, anxiously trying to reassure him about the safety and authenticity of the vaccine that he had sent him:

> "By the conveyance which brings you this, you will . . . receive vaccine matter, such as I employ with my patients here . . . the virus you began to inoculate with came from my stock, and . . . with a continuation of the same, I am now, almost daily, inoculating children in the metropolis . . . it . . . is from that stock I am using among all my patients here . . . The whole is from my original stock."[235]

The resupplied vaccine was used in America with much greater success than the first supply: President Jefferson wrote an account of how he used it, along with his sons-in-law, on two hundred people, and "two or three only had from two to half a dozen pustules on the inoculated arm, and nowhere else."[236] This was the same proportion and type of pustular cases that Pearson and Woodville were achieving with the more attenuated form of their vaccine; Waterhouse had at first unwittingly selected a more virulent strain of the virus when he selected matter from a pustule other than at the site of injection — with the second supply of the same stock of vaccine, he took matter only from the primary tumour and advised those whom he supplied with vaccine to do likewise. However, even with this precaution, the new supply of vaccine still continued occasionally to produce symptoms; for example,

Dr. Shore of Petersburg wrote to Waterhouse on the 27th November, 1802:

> ". . . With the vaccine virus you sent here, our physicians commenced their inoculation early in the Spring . . . in one instance it was said to be attended with a pretty numerous eruption, and in another to have excited a violent disease, attended with fever, in a person who had undergone the small-pox."[237]

Waterhouse was of course unfortunate, like Pearson in the Petworth incident, to have previously been the victim of an unpredictable resurgence of virulence in the virus. Most vaccinators had experienced some cases with pustular eruptions, but usually these were not severe. However, the general problem of the virus reverting back to a more virulent form was by no means rare; Jenner, in a letter written in March, 1801 to Waterhouse, came near to admitting this:

> "Now I conceive that at some period of your inoculation, which may now have escaped your recollection, an imperfect pustule arose, either from some peculiarity in the constitution of your patient, or some alteration in the qualities of your matter, and that from this stock you propagated. The consequence was, that continued degeneracy you complain of in the nature of the disease. The same thing has happened to many in this country, and indeed many other parts of Europe. Now either from an idiosyncracy, or some change in the nature of the virus, a variety has sprung up in the character of the pustule. The practitioners not deeply versed in the nature of cow pox has inadvertently inoculated from this variety. He proceeds with his inoculation hoping to call back his original pustule, but alas! In vain."[238]

This is a remarkably accurate description of what had happened to Waterhouse as far as it goes; all that is missing is the fact that the "imperfect pustule" was an eruptive pustule of smallpox — and the rest of facts of the situation then fall into place. (Jenner was wrong, however, not being able to attenuate this "spurious" disease — this was achieved by Woodville and Pearson through arm-to-arm inoculation.)

Jenner's admission that Waterhouse's experience was similar to that of some practitioners in England has already been discussed, and in general terms, it is a conclusion that is substantially correct — although it was rare for the virus to reach the level of virulence that it did in the Boston area.

CHAPTER 7

Vaccination on the Continent of Europe

The experience of vaccinators outside of Britain and America appears to have been very much the same as that already discussed. Evidence on this is much more difficult to find in English libraries for obvious reasons, but reports did appear in contemporary medical journals and letters which enable us to tentatively examine the nature of vaccines used abroad. Often these reports are no more of a hint of what might be uncovered through further research; for example, Baron mentions in his biography of Jenner that the latter sent some of his vaccine to his friend John Clinch, practising in Newfoundland, and according to a report in December, 1800, there were "some untoward circumstances which occurred among those who were first vaccinated at Portugal Cove."[239] No indication is given as to what these were, but it is not hard to imagine what these might have been, but only research into local source materials would settle this question. Sometimes considerable detail is available on the symptomatic results of the use of vaccines, but it is not entirely clear whether the vaccine in question came from Jenner or Woodville/Pearson. H. M. Husson, in his review of the Continental literature of vaccination in 1801, gives detailed accounts of the different kinds of eruption experienced by European practitioners: "eruptions 'rosacées', eruptions 'miliares' and some variolous-like eruptions. The eruption 'rosacée' consists of red spots on different parts of the body."[240] Husson states that these eruptions were experienced almost universally, and he mentions by name Dr. Odier of Geneva, Dr. Aubert of Paris, Dr. Sacco of Milan, Dr. Scassi at Gènes, and Dr. De Carro at Vienna, as having experienced "spurious vaccine."[241] Reports were made by the relevant medical authorities at Geneva, Paris, Rheims and elsewhere which detailed the kinds of eruptions experienced.[242] If the English vaccinators were confused about the results of their work, one can imagine the problems that other medical practitioners had in explaining the effects of their inoculations. In some cases, Continental doctors had come to England to learn the new techniques and methods, and had gone back home carrying a supply of smallpox virus with them under the new name of cowpox vaccine. For example, Dr. Aubert had spent some time in the London Smallpox Hospital working with Woodville, and had subsequently returned to practice in Paris; he had some difficulty in propagating the new vaccine, and Woodville spent some weeks in France inoculating the "new" disease — and as this seems to have formed the basis of the main stock of French vaccine, it is not surprising that Aubert in his report on vaccination found that "the vaccine . . . manifested on all parts of the body vesicular pustules . . ."[243] Husson does mention one instance of a supply of vaccine coming from Jenner: "Dr. Odier, who had received from Jenner some thread impregnated with vaccine obtained at Geneva spurious vaccine, in his first attempt at vaccination."[244] Odier in his own reports on vaccination, mentioned the whole range of different kinds of eruption; but appears to have experienced particularly the eruptions 'miliares': "they are very small pimples . . . never suppurating . . ."[245] Orthodox smallpox pustules were also observed, but these were explained as being the result of natural smallpox infection resulting from an epidemic.[246] However, Waterhouse claimed that "the case at Geneva, under Dr. Odier, was ours exactly"[247] and Ring, in reviewing Odier's report on his experiences, expressed surprise at some of his conclusions:

> "One opinion advanced by our author, appears rather singular. He says, 'It appears certain, that the inoculated Cow-pox is as much milder than the inoculated small-pox, as the latter is milder than the natural small-pox, at least in the three first years of life: **for after the age of three years there is no great difference between the mildness of the Cow-pox and the inoculated small-Pox**'."[248]

Ring went on to note that Odier reported "eruptions resembling the smallpox . . . in about two to three cases in every hundred; and in one or two instances, the eruption was very abundant; but it appeared evidently to be owing to the epidemic smallpox then prevailing."[249] Without a much more careful scrutiny of the original evidence it is impossible to properly evaluate the latter interpretation, but given what we know about the nature of vaccines at this time, and Odier's general account of the severity of the disease above three-year-olds, it is likely that these smallpox pustular eruptions were a result of the vaccine itself.

Jenner later denied the charge that it was his stock of vaccine that had been responsible for Odier's experiences of pustules in Geneva,[250] although he produced no evidence one way or the other to refute this claim. One major instance of Jenner's vaccine producing pustular eruptions which he did not dispute, was the experience of Danish vaccinators. In the summer of 1801, Jenner sent vaccine via his friend Marcet to Dr. Winslow, Professor of Medicine in Copenhagen; by the 19th December of the same year, 705 vaccinations had been carried out with this supply.[251] A special committee was set up by the Government to study vaccination, and direct observations were made on 297 cases, most of which had been carried out by Winslow. The committee reported that:

> "A few vaccinated have eight or ten days after inoculation, caught the small-pox, but the committee attributes this only to a prior infection before the vaccine has taken effect."[252]

The fact that the incubation period for inoculated smallpox would fall approximately in the eight to ten days range, would make one a little suspicious of this result, and a subsequent Government report stated unambiguously that vaccination was in fact a "pustular disease". Jenner wrote to Marcet in February, 1803, and discussed his own interpretation of this finding:

> "The Copenhagen Report on the subject of Vaccination is equally satisfactory with that of other Countries. Nevertheless it strikes me that the Virus they employ there, has probably undergone some change . . . for it is said in the Report, 'those inoculated, frequently have Eruptions' . . . Similar occurrences to those in Denmark, have taken place both in this Country and many others. In Hanover the same thing took place and in a District in Scotland . . . The

origin of this Deviation in my opinion is this — the use of the Vaccine Fluid when taken so late from a Pustule, that it was **beginning** to undergo a change which rendered it incapable of exciting the same effect precisely as if it had been taken at an early period. The truth of this theory seems to have been exemplified in many instances . . ."[253]

There is of course no reason to believe from the viewpoint of current virological and medical knowledge, that the timing of taking virus would have the significant effects postulated by Jenner (and some of his contemporaries, such as Pearson, claimed from their experience, that the timing of taking the vaccine made no difference whatsoever to the effects produced). Once again, the conclusion is inescapable: pustules resulted from the practice of early vaccination, because the vaccines employed were derived from smallpox and not cowpox.

CHAPTER 8

The Attenuation of Smallpox Virus

The question to arise out of the previous review of the historical evidence on the nature of the early vaccines is, how was the attenuation of the strain of smallpox originating in Woodville's patients achieved? Woodville's own lymph employed in the London Smallpox Hospital was not discontinued until 1836, for according to Dr. George Gregory, who was physician to the hospital in the 1830s:

> "On the 20th January, 1799, cow pock was found in Mr. Harrison's dairy, in Gray's Inn Lane, from which source, Dr. Woodville, my predecessor at the Small Pox Hospital, commenced a series of vaccinations. That same stock remained in use up to the year 1836."[254]

This prolonged use of the first vaccines appears to have been very common, as was seen with the continuation of Jenner's original stock well into the 1840's, and Woodville's lymph both in the hospital and outside of it. Bousquet stated that it was used in Paris down to 1836,[255] and Steinbrenner — his father had received vaccine from Woodville in 1802 — was still using it in 1840.[256] Similarly, De Carro mentioned in a letter to Monro in 1825, that he was still using (and he had been responsible for distributing vaccine to many parts of the world) lymph derived from British and Milanese sources in 1799.[257] These vaccines were only abandoned in the late 1830s and 1840s on the grounds that they had become so weakened by arm-to-arm passage that they were no longer giving significant protection against attacks of smallpox,[258] presumably through inadequate stimulation of the antibody response. Moore in his *History of Vaccination* claimed that pustular cases were eliminated by ensuring that "vaccine lymph alone was employed",[259] and this explanation both does and does not fit the historical evidence. Inasmuch as virtually all the early vaccines were derived from smallpox, to talk about the selection of "vaccine lymph" (i.e. vaccine derived from cowpox) does not make sense; but given that all the early vaccinators recognised the importance of taking lymph from the tumour at the site of injection, which classically was meant to be the sole eruptive symptom of vaccination, there are reasons to believe (as we have seen, for example, with Woodville's experience) that this was of some importance.

A careful reading of the historical literature reveals, in fact, that several different variolators had been able to attenuate smallpox virus through arm-to-arm passage of the kind employed by the vaccinators. The first publication to make reference to the mild effects achieved by taking virus from a previous site of inoculation was J. Z. Holwell's book on variolation in India, published in 1767. The Indian inoculators always used "matter from the inoculated pustules of the previous year", with the result that "a few pustules generally appear round the edge of the wound . . . without a single eruption on any other part of the body."[260] The following year, Angelo Gatti's book on inoculation was published in English, and among the many shrewd and sound comments on smallpox and the practice of variolation, was a note on the question of attenuation:

> "I have long suspected, that the variolous matter became milder by inoculation; and consequently, that a repetition of the like operations would render it still more harmless, though not less efficacious. This conjecture is now become a truth, from the experiments I have tried, and those which were made in England by the most experienced inoculators."[261]

Unfortunately, as far as I am aware, Gatti never published details of his experiments, and it is not even entirely clear whether he selected virus for inoculation from the sites of previous inoculations, or whether he merely selected virus from eruptive pustules of inoculated cases (it was almost certainly the former). The English inoculators that he referred to were probably the Sutton family and their associates, who had pioneered a return to safer methods of variolation during the 1760s.

There has been some misunderstanding about the

method of inoculation adopted by the Suttons; as they attempted on financial grounds to keep their innovation a secret, it was rather difficult for contemporaries to discover the reasons for their success. All the early reports in the years 1766 and 1767 however, unanimously agreed that the Suttons at the beginning of their practice took virus early from the site of a previous inoculation,[262] but it was soon claimed that experience showed that there was no difference in effect between this virus and that selected from an eruptive pustule of a case of natural smallpox.[263] In 1768, the apologist and propagandist for the Sutton family, the Rev. R. Houlton, categorically denied that their success was the result of taking virus early from the site of a previous inoculation,[264] and quoted from a pamphlet by Dr. Giles Watts to support his case:

> "I . . . (have) seen a **great number** of persons inoculated in the new way with well concocted yellow matter, taken from the natural, as well as from the inoculated small-pox, all of whom have had the distemper full as lightly as those, who have been inoculated with crude variolous lymph (i.e., matter taken early from the site of a previous inoculation)."[265]

In 1767, Bromfield published a pamphlet summarising an experiment in which a series of patients was inoculated with virus from previous inoculated cases, and twenty children inoculated with matter of "the fourteenth in descent, from the natural sort first inoculated", had the disease in the usual way — "Some of them had the disease very mild, and others rather severe . . ."[266] Bromfield did not make it clear whether virus was taken from the **sites of previous inoculations,** or whether it was merely taken from the eruptive pustules of inoculated cases. As he seemed to have been unaware of the importance of this distinction, and did not even mention it, it is likely that virus was taken at random from inoculated cases, and therefore mainly from eruptive pustules. Although some inoculators at this time were denying that virus taken from the sites of inoculation produced milder results than that taken from elsewhere, it should be realised that these conclusions were completely impressionistic, and had not been based on

serial arm-to-arm passage of one strain of virus systematically selected from previous sites of injection.

That the question of the effects of using virus from sites of previous injection had not been settled by contemporaries, was indicated by Mudge, in his discussion in 1777 of an experiment involving this type of virus. After noting that some inoculators had explained the success of the Suttons through their use of virus from the inoculation site, Mudge warned against the latter practice on the grounds that it was not a sure mode of protecting patients against future attacks of smallpox. He described the first part of the experiment as follows:

> "Messrs. Longworthy and Arscott, surgeons, in the spring of 1776, inoculated at Plympton, a neighbouring town [to Plymouth], forty patients; of which number, thirty were injected with crude matter from the arm of a young woman [from the site of inoculation], five days after she had been inoculated with concocted matter, which did eventually produce in her a pretty smart fever, and a sufficient number of eruptions. The other ten were inoculated with matter of another kind, which I procured, in a concocted state, from a pustule of the natural smallpox. The arm of all the forty patients took the injection; and the latter ten, after the eruptive fever, had the [inoculated] smallpox in the usual way. Of the other thirty, though the injection took place, so as to inflame them considerably, and to produce a very large prominent pustule, with matter on it, in each of them, yet not one of them had eruptive fever, or a single subsequent eruption, on any part of the body . . . It is to be remarked too that the matter which was in those pustules having been used to inoculate others produced on them exactly the same appearances, unattended also with either fever or smallpox."[267]

Mudge goes on to describe how the thirty patients with just a local pustule at the site of injection were again inoculated, but this time with concocted matter taken after the eruptive fever. All thirty were infected and "had smallpox in different degrees, but in the usual way of inoculated patients."[268] Mudge concluded that concocted matter was necessary for certain inoculated infection of patients, and that the single local pustule resulting from the use of early virus selected from sites of inoculation, did not ensure protection from future attacks of smallpox. However, Mudge did not state the period between the first and second inoculations, and if this was less than ten days, the "success" of the second inoculations is not entirely surprising. But the important point to emerge out of these experiments for the present paper, is that Mudge and his colleagues were able to produce a local pustule at the site of injection, without pustular eruptions elsewhere, and were able to propagate this attenuated form of virus through inoculation, to a further group of patients. Almost identical results were achieved by John Covey, an apothecary at Basingstoke, in a similar experiment in 1787 — of nine people inoculated with virus from a site of previous inoculation, only two had pustules other than at the site of injection.[269]

Although these experiments were producing purely local reactions through the use of virus from the site of inoculation, it is clear from earlier accounts of inoculators experimenting with what they thought was the Suttonian method of inoculation, that this was not always the case. Dimsdale explicitly stated that his experience with such virus was identical to that selected from the eruptive pustules of natural smallpox,[270] and Chandler who appears at least in his early practice to have relied almost exclusively on virus from the site of injection, obviously had pustular cases, although the proportion was unclear. Chandler claimed that his patients had:

> "without one exception gone through the disease so very slightly, as scarce ever to have been sick; not one of them had been obliged to keep within doors, or how longer than is usual than a perfect state of health; not one of them has had an equivocal eruption, though some few of them has had no other appearance than that on the punctured arm; and the fullest patient has not had a number exceeding two hundred pustules."[271]

We must therefore conclude that although Mudge and colleagues, and Covey, were producing merely a local reaction with virus from the site of inoculation, other inoculators experienced a much more heterogeneous range of symptoms with the same kind of virus. Perhaps this should not surprise us, as the modern practice of the attenuation of viruses involves multiple serial passage. It is likely therefore, that the radical attenuation of smallpox would have been achieved only through similar multiple passage, involving the arm-to-arm inoculation of a particular strain of virus.

In 1799, Salmade published a treatise on variolation which included a discussion of the effects of using virus taken from a natural case as against an inoculated case of smallpox. He quoted an experiment by Goetz which had found that a succession of twenty inoculations using matter from a previous inoculation, appeared to have no influence on the result of the ensuing disease. Like Bromfield, however, Salmade did not indicate whether virus was taken from the site of previous inoculation or from a pustule of an inoculated case; he referred to a belief amongst some French doctors, that a succession of inoculated cases would weaken the virus to a point of nullity, to the extent that it would be without effect when used in inoculation.[272] As no details are given of the evidence on which these conclusions were based, it is impossible to evaluate their significance. Nine years later, Adams published an account of experiments at the London Smallpox Hospital, deliberately designed to transform smallpox through arm-to-arm inoculation into vaccine. He was particularly concerned to obtain a tumour at the site of injection similar to that of vaccination, and claimed great success in this objective:

> "By continuing with great caution to inoculate at the hospital from Pearl Small Pox [a mild form of smallpox], and afterwards by selecting those arms which had the most appearance of Cow Pox, we at last succeeded in procuring a succession of arms so nearly resembling the vaccine, that an universal suspicion prevailed among the parents, that they were deceived by the substitution of one for the other."[273]

It is not clear how far Adams managed to eliminate pustular eruptions in the later cases, as he was more concerned to discuss the character of the tumour than other symptoms of the inoculations. He did, however, publish a small section of the hospital register to illustrate the nature of his results, and from this it does appear that arm-to-arm inoculation using a site of previous injection did radically attenuate the virus being used. For example, on the 14th August, 1805, William Croft was inoculated from the person suffering from the mild case of natural smallpox, and had 150 pustules; from Croft, on the 26th August, Rogers was inoculated, with a result that it "was perfectly vaccine in all its stages". On 2nd September, Mary Ann Dobins was "inoculated from Rogers" and "the arm proved vaccine in all its stages":

> "From Dobins, seven were inoculated; of these, five had no eruptions, the arms were vaccine in all the stages, and in the appearance of the scab. One had a perfectly vaccine appearance on the arm, areola, and brown scab, [but] with one hundred variolous pustules . . . The other had a vaccine arm somewhat irregular, with fever, but no pustules. From the last, were inoculated four. Of these, two had vaccine arms, perfect in all their stages, and without pustules. One had the vaccine regular, excepting that the edges sloped in such a manner, that the base was broader than the apex . . . The other had small pustules . . ."[274]

Adams did not always specify whether virus was taken from the site of a previous inoculation, and in the earlier cases, whether there were pustular eruptions or not, but as he himself stated that he was "selecting those arms which had the most appearance of Cow Pox", we can assume that he was taking material from tumours at the site of injection that most resembled vaccination. He did, however, specifically mention taking virus from eruptive pustules on particular occasions, and found, as Woodville had done before him, that this produced significantly severer results:

> "From Stevens fluid was taken from both the arm and the pustules to inoculate others. The fluid from the arm produced the vaccine vesicle, though in a few instances attended with secondary vesicles. The fluid from the

> pustules produced true small pox pustular cases for three successions."[275]

The main series of trial inoculations amounted to "at least two or three hundred"[276] but Adams's work was severely hampered by the current hostility of parents to vaccination, and their demand that "their own children had unequivocal symptoms of Small Pox."[277] However, in the preface to his book, Adams stated that in the "five calendar months" that had elapsed since the beginning of the series of inoculations described, "nothing has occurred but the same uniform effects from successive inoculations."[278] His overall conclusion was that "the facts are . . . sufficient to show that we were hasty in determining that the kind of smallpox matter used for inoculation, was unimportant."[279]

After a period of initial hostility — Jenner at first implacably rejected Adams's findings — contemporaries came to accept his work; Baron, for example, stated that Adams had "succeeded in producing a benign form of variola attended with scarcely any eruption of pustules and little or no constitutional affection; this species of smallpox he considered capable of being rendered fixed and permanent."[280] In fact, Baron himself believed that smallpox could be radically attenuated through arm-to-arm passage, and quoted Jenner in support of this view:

> "After a series of inoculations with true variolous matter it has often been observed that the severity of the symptoms and the number of pustules gradually diminish till only **one** is to be seen, at the point of insertion . . . This fact did not escape the observation of Dr. Jenner; in reference to which he has remarked in one of his memoranda, 'Here then we see the cowpox and the smallpox acting similar parts: and that in either case the virus may steal, as it were, imperceptibly through the constitution, and give no signal of its presence'."[281]

The next attempt to transform variola into vaccine through arm-to-arm inoculation took place in France at the end of 1826 and beginning of 1827. M. Guillon, an old navy surgeon, wrote two letters to a medical colleague, describing his work, which were abstracted in one of the French medical journals:

> "This practitioner announces, that having no vaccine virus during a very fatal small-pox epidemic, he took on the 17th of December, 1826, **some variolous matter** from a girl fifteen years of age, **on the fifth day of eruption,** and he inserted it in ten places on the arm of a healthy infant still at the breast. This inoculation, M. Guillon says, produced ten beautiful **vaccine vesicles,** with which, on the ninth day, forty-two infants were inoculated, under the eyes of the local authorities: these furnished virus for the inoculation of one hundred, who were inoculated on the 3rd of January, in the presence of the magistrates and many medical men. In a second letter, dated the 16th of January, 1827, he observes: 'The numerous vaccinations [inoculations with variolous matter] effected since my discovery, confirm more and more the perfect identity of the variolous with the vaccine virus . . . Every point in which matter is inserted proceeds well, and in their intervals in many individuals an eruption of variolous pustules takes place, and produces fever'."[282]

Guillon's work appears to have been stopped by the local magistrates on the grounds of potential hazards of spreading smallpox from such inoculations. Guillon does not seem to have had a very clear idea of how he was achieving attenuated effects; the purely local response on the infant at the breast was presumably a function of partial antibody immunity acquired from the mother, but subsequent modifications must have been the result of arm-to-arm inoculations, using the sites of previous injections as the source of virus. The key point in all the inoculations which produced attenuated forms of smallpox in the post-vaccination period, was that they were conducted in the belief that the vaccine should always be selected from the purely local site of injection. One other important point to emerge out of Guillon's account, was the eruption of secondary pustules on the arms in the areas of the sites of inoculation; as we have seen, this was a feature of many of the more attenuated forms of inoculation made with Woodville's lymph and was characteristic of other instances of the attenuation of smallpox virus through arm-to-arm inoculation at a relatively early stage.

A more informed transformation of smallpox into vaccine was undertaken by a German surgeon, Dr. Basil Thiele of Kazan, in 1839. He showed a good understanding of the historical literature on attenuation procedures:

> "From the history of the inoculation of natural smallpox I knew, on the one hand, that the reinoculation of inoculated smallpox first tried by Professor Gatti at Pisa in 1763 makes their progress milder, and that there were examples of fifteen hundred consecutive inoculation experiments without harmful consequences . . ."[283]

What the statement on the fifteen hundred consecutive inoculation experiments referred to is unclear; I have not been able to trace in Gatti's published writings an account of such a series, but this may be a function of the unavailability of the relevant literature in England. Thiele went on to quote a further unfamiliar reference: "Dr. Robert in Marseilles found that if smallpox is inoculated with milk, it can cause only local pustules, and he derives vaccine from this."[284] Again, we can only assume that Robert was practising arm-to-arm inoculation, but this would have to be checked against original information if and where it could be located. Thiele described his own derivation of vaccine from variola as follows:

> ". . . my objective was crowned with complete success . . . a perfect vaccine was formed from the inoculatory matter after nine inoculated generations; if one deviated during the second and third generation from the prescribed path, it did not happen altogether rarely that smallpox broke out all over the body, which it was possible to reduce again to vaccine . . . several hundred cases [were involved] . . . Regarding the reduction of smallpox to vaccine, the lymph from smallpox must lie first of all for ten days between sheets of glass which are stuck down with wax, and then it must be thinned down with cow's

> milk and inoculated like ordinary vaccine; this inoculation forms big pocks in the inoculated place, and the high temperature occurring only once with ordinary vaccination, occurs twice . . . and sometimes pocks come into being not only in the inoculated place but also in its neighbourhood, but they are always quite small . . . This procedure must be observed for ten generations, and gradually the pock becomes just like the vaccine . . . Later experiences have shown that the consecutive high temperature fails to appear already in the fifth generation, and then . . . the immediate transfer from arm to arm [without dilution with cow's milk] can take place."[285]

The procedure of diluting smallpox matter with cow's milk cannot but provoke a wry smile, but although Thiele's methods now appear to us to be amusing, he did make some very sound observations on the attenuating process. Firstly, he recognised that it was not a simple linear process, and that there were somewhat unpredictable resurgences of virulence in the virus. Secondly, he discovered that it took serial passage of at least ten generations before the virus had begun to adopt the approximate characteristics of conventional vaccine material. And thirdly, he noted that although the eruption of pocks became localised, there were satellite eruptions, at least in the initial phases of attenuation, in the area of the site of inoculation. There is no indication of whether this vaccine of Thiele's was put into regular use, but as he had derived it (along with another vaccine derived from the inoculation of smallpox on to the udders of a cow) because of dissatisfaction with the quality of conventional vaccine, it is likely that it was adopted as a standard lymph.

The last example of the use of smallpox as a direct source of vaccine has a somewhat more modern ring. The renowned French clinician, A. Trousseau, described in 1869 how he had resorted to variolation because of the unavailability of conventional vaccine, and the results of his attempts at attenuating the virus through arm-to-arm inoculation:

> ". . . I proceeded with a view to communicate the disease in as mild a form as possible . . . I asked myself . . .

> whether by successive series of inoculations in the human subject, an equally great modification of the disease [smallpox] could be produced as had been produced in the sheep [with tag-sore], by which the eruption had been limited to a single pustule in the spot where the inoculation had been made. I tried the experiment at the Necker Hospital . . . We obtained the desired result in some children, to the extent that the mother pustule, the master pimple **(le maitre bouton)**, the pustule of inoculation was alone developed, and that around it there were little pustules, its satellites. If we could be sure of always attaining equally fortunate results, inoculation ought to be the rule, for then it would be attended by no risk, and its consequences would be purely beneficial . . . Unfortunately, matters did not turn out so propitiously. In some cases, I attained complete success of having only the pustule of inoculation; but in others, in which the very same virus had been employed, there were general eruptions, and, worse still, communication of small-pox to non-inoculated persons. In one case, regarding which I shall have to speak in connection with the subject of vaccine virus, the small-pox resumed all its original violence, after having passed through a succession of individuals in a series of inoculations. This result is opposed to those recorded by the inoculators, who made out that the variolous virus becomes progressively milder as the succession of transplantations proceeds."[286]

Trousseau did not make it clear what his method of attenuating his virus was, but as in the modification of tag-sore in sheep, the inoculator "took virus from one in which the symptoms were mildest,"[287] and he emphasised the importance of achieving a single pustule at the site of inoculation, it is likely that he was taking virus from the site of inoculation in the mildest of cases. One major point stands out in his account: the flaring of virulence of the virus, even after having achieved successful attenuation to the degree of producing just a local pustule. This, to some extent, echoed Thiele's experience, but the true parallel is with the resurgence of virulence with

Pearson's vaccine in Petworth, and Jenner's in Marblehead. Ironically, Pearson, Woodville, Jenner and the other early vaccinators all persisted with their strain of attenuated smallpox in the belief that it had derived from cowpox, and after two years or so, these attenuated strains appeared to have achieved complete stability (there were no reports of resurgence of virulence after the initial year or so).

CHAPTER 9

The Virology of Smallpox Attenuation

Having reviewed all the historical evidence on the attenuation of smallpox virus through arm-to-arm inoculation, we must now consider whether the findings of current laboratory research into the virology of pox viruses can account for the findings of the historical literature. This obviously raises technical questions which can only be answered by a qualified virologist, but it is possible to discuss the findings of this book at a hypothetical level. The first major point to note is that the relationship between smallpox, cowpox and current strains of vaccinia has not been settled by modern virological research. While cowpox and vaccinia are similar in their fairly wide host range and growth characteristics, in tissue culture variola is more like vaccinia than is cowpox, with regard to cytoplasmic inclusions and general serological characteristics; ceiling temperatures in the chick embryo and the nature of the lesions on the chorioallantois after three days is different for each one of the three viruses, although they share an identical morphological structure.[288] The three viruses are very closely related in their basic characteristics, but differences have made it impossible to establish any clear-cut genealogical relationship between them. The differences are sufficiently great for Herrlich and his colleagues to have questioned whether vaccinia has been derived from either smallpox or cowpox,[289] but this notion arising out of laboratory studies is so obviously contradicted by the evidence on the historical origin of the virus, that it clearly must be in error. One of the problems is that the viruses vary so significantly **within** the three categories of classification, that definite conclusions appear, at least at this stage, very difficult to reach. If laboratory research cannot solve this question, can the historical evidence? The problem here is that although there is no doubt that vaccinia was originally derived from either smallpox or cowpox, it is not clear which particular virus was involved in the origination of current strains. Almost from the beginning of the nineteenth century, there was controversy about the relationship between the various viruses:

many workers in the field claimed to have transformed smallpox into cowpox through the inoculation of the cow, but the most recent attempts to achieve this under modern laboratory conditions have failed.[290] Some virologists have therefore argued that the successful transformation of smallpox into cowpox was a function of the inadequate safeguards against secondary contamination of cows with vaccinia virus kept in the research establishments where the variolation of cows was being attempted.[291] However, many of the later workers were aware of possible contamination, and went to some lengths to guard against this possibility,[292] but more important is the large number of claimed successful transformations under conditions which would not be likely to give rise to secondary infection. An example of this is the work of Badcock; he was a chemist living in Brighton and had suffered a severe attack of smallpox at the end of 1836, a few months after having been re-vaccinated.[293] This failure of the current strain of vaccine led him, like many of his contemporaries to seek a more effective supply and in December, 1840, he began a series of experiments involving the inoculation of cows with smallpox virus. According to Copeman, Badcock performed in the following twenty-five years "more than five hundred variolous inoculations", of which only thirty-eight were successful.[294] Badcock's vaccine was used very extensively: "he supplied it to hundreds of medical practitioners, and many thousands of children are said to have been successfully vaccinated with it."[295] As he had set up a special stable for his inoculation experiments, and he was operating at a time when most supplies of vaccine had been derived from Woodville's strain of attenuated smallpox, it is difficult to see how under such conditions secondary infection with vaccinia virus derived from cowpox, could have taken place. The relatively small proportion of successful transformations — about 7½ per cent — would mean that only very large series such as Badcock's, could expect any degree of success. The major problem with transforming variola into vaccina through cow inoculations, is that the mechanism of transformation has never been understood, and successful outcomes have very much been hit-or-miss affairs.

Similar problems have been encountered by virologists attempting to transform cowpox into strains of virus which resemble currently used types of vaccinia virus.[296] In the way that there is a considerable body of historical evidence for the use of smallpox as the source of vaccine (either directly through arm-to-arm attenuation as demonstrated in this book, or indirectly through the inoculation of cows), there is similar evidence for the use of genuine cowpox strains as the basis of vaccines. We have seen that the Kentish Town cowpox lymph and a strain of horsepox was used by Jenner and others on a restricted basis, and after about 1838 there is no doubt that Estlin, Ceely and others began to use other genuine strains of cowpox as the source of their vaccine.[297] Since that time, both cowpox and smallpox appeared to have been used; the present strain of vaccine used in England (at the Lister Institute) is said to have originated "from a Prussian soldier with smallpox in the war of 1870."[298] (Although there is no firm evidence for this.) When it was received in this country in 1907, it was, however, in the form of calf lymph well adapted to the calf, and all vaccines have been passaged in non-human hosts since the end of the nineteenth century. This means that modern virological research into the characteristics of current strains of vaccinia cannot resolve the problem raised by this book: the nature of a vaccine derived from the attenuation of smallpox, through arm-to-arm inoculation in an exclusively human host. However, the findings of contemporary virology on the attenuation and adaptation of viruses to particular organic environments obviously have a relevance to the construction of hypotheses which might be capable of explaining the historical findings.

In 1928, J. C. G. Ledingham and D. McClean published a paper which demonstrated that vaccine virus propagated in the rabbit dermis through serial passage, led to enhanced potency of the virus for the dermis, but "a loss of propagating power on scarification surfaces,"[299] i.e. virus adapted to grow in the dermis, lost its capacity to grow effectively on the skin surface. Ledingham and McClean were unable to explain this result, but it is clear from this and other work that viruses are capable of adapting themselves to specific areas of the body, losing their capacity to effectively reproduce themselves in other areas where critical conditions for growth are absent. In the case of the attenuation of smallpox through arm-to-arm inoculation, the virus was systematically selected from the site of a previous inoculation, where it would have grown under very different conditions to those viruses in body pustules, which would have all experienced a systematic body reaction, including blood-borne transmission. In this situation, drawing an analogy from Ledingham and McClean's work, virus from sites of inoculation would have become adapted to grow at the skin surface in epithelial cells, and would lose their capacity for systematic body growth and virulence for the total organism. This process of adaptation would consist of the natural selection of mutants efficient for growing in a particular organic environment, involving the transformation of the genotype.

The above hypothesis does not specify what the critical body environmental conditions were for the attenuation of smallpox virus. Work on the pox viruses during the last twenty years or so has shown that temperature is one of the critical conditions for growth, and that there is some relationship between the virulence of a virus and the ceiling temperature at which it will grow in various cell environments. This is not a simple one-to-one relationship: although it was originally thought that ceiling temperature was a good laboratory test for discriminating between variola major and variola minor, with the former virulent virus having a higher ceiling temperature than the latter much less virulent type, and subsequent work on intermediate African strains seemed to confirm this overall relationship, very recent research has thrown into question the validity of using ceiling temperatures as a measure of the natural virulence of smallpox viruses.[300] (The whole notion of a basic distinction between variola major and variola minor has also been brought into question by recent work.[301]) Baxby, however, has found a possible relationship between the human pathogenicity of various smallpox vaccines and their capacity to grow at elevated temperatures on the chick chorioallantois.[302]

More directly relevant to the findings of this book, is the work of Kirn and Braunwald on the attenuation of vaccinia virus through the selection of cold variants in serial passage at regularly decreasing temperatures. The wild vaccinia strain WR underwent 10 transfers at 30°C, 4 transfers at 29°, one transfer at 27° and 5 transfers at 25°, representing a total of 20 transfers; an identical strain was subjected to 21 transfers in the same condition of culture on KB cells, but at a constant temperature of 37°C, to act as a control in the measurement of virulence characteristics. Kirn and Braunwald were successful at producing a cold variant, which became very much less virulent than either the original or control strain (which was unaffected by serial passage at constant temperature), and summarised their findings as follows:

> ". . . By means of transfers at regularly decreasing temperatures, a cold variant developing at 25°C has been selected . . . The cold variant has completely lost its virulence in mice by the intracerebral route, and its intradermal infectivity in rabbits is 41 times weaker than that of the wild virus . . ."[303]

Kirn and Braunwald go on to point out that similar findings have been made with the polio and encéphalmyélocardite viruses, and conclude that the phenomena of virus sensitivity to temperature might be a general one.[304] No attempt has ever been made to produce a cold variant of variola through serial passage at decreasing temperatures, but given the similarity of the vaccinia and variola viruses (the former in many cases being derived from the latter), and the finding of a general relationship between the loss of virulence and the production of cold variants, it is likely that a cold variant of smallpox with a loss of virulence is possible. Griffith has recently summarised experience with the attenuation of a number of different viruses:

> "Most of the virus strains used in the production of currently available vaccines have been recently developed by subjecting a natural virus isolate to various attenuating procedures such as repeated subculture at low temperatures and adapting it to grow profusely in tissue cells of a

type which do not readily support growth of the freshly isolated virulent organism. These procedures have been successfully applied in the development of measles, mumps and rubella vaccines."[305]

Applying these findings to smallpox vaccines, it might be hypothesised that the early vaccines were derived through arm-to-arm inoculation of smallpox (repeated subculture) at low temperature, whereas later vaccines originated from the growth of the virus (smallpox) in tissue cells which do not readily support growth (in the cow).

The historical evidence certainly points to the importance of reduced temperature in producing the attenuated effects of inoculated smallpox. Holwell noted in his account of Indian variolation that:

> ". . . early on the morning succeeding the operation, four collons [an earthen pot containing about two gallons] of cold water are ordered to be thrown over the patient, from the head downwards, and to be repeated every morning and evening until the fever comes on . . . [and] then to desist until the appearance of the eruptions . . . and then to pursue the cold bathing as before, through the course of the disease, and until the scabs of the pustules drop off . . . Confinement to the house is absolutely forbid, and the inoculated are ordered to be exposed to every air that blows . . ."[306]

Gatti conducted an experiment which can be interpreted as evidence in favour of the temperature/virulence hypothesis:

> ". . . I desired two of my patients inoculated in the hand, to hold it in cold water as often and long as possible, from the first appearance of the local eruption to that of the fever. In both cases, the fever came on; but it was hardly perceptible, and lasted but four or five hours . . . an inoculated patient, treated according to the foregoing rules, during the first period, will have hardly any fever in the next, and certainly a very slight eruption, and perhaps none at all."[307]

One of the innovations of the Sutton family in their highly

successful practice of variolation, was what was known as the "cold method"; Sydenham in the previous century had advocated the exposure of patients suffering from natural smallpox to the fresh air, and during the summer "to cool them . . . by rising and wearing very thin clothes"[308] and the Suttons took over this policy in their inoculation practice.[309] Thomas Christie, in his account of smallpox in Ceylon, claimed that the higher temperature in that Island, and the adjoining continent of India, meant that variolation in general was less successful than it was in European countries:

> ". . . the number of Inoculated Patients [in Ceylon between the 1st October, 1800 and the 30th September, 1802] amounted to 4,158, of which number 108 died, being nearly 1 in 38 . . . it is probable that under no circumstances, could the practice be more successfully conducted amongst the adults in that Island, where the thermometer is seldom so low as 70°, and in general many degrees higher. The Variolous inoculation by European Surgeons, in most parts of India, has been chiefly confined to the children of European Parents, and from every information I have been enabled to procure, it is conceived that not less than one in forty of these died. Dr. Fleming, the distinguished head of the Medical Department in Bengal, has, I am told calculated the mortality at a still higher rate, and conceives that nearly one in thirty of the children of Europeans, inoculated with Smallpox at Calcutta, died. I am aware, that it has been said, that the proportion of deaths from inoculation by the itinerant Brahmins in Bengal, has been very small indeed, and as they avail themselves of the cold seasons for their operations . . . I can readily believe that the mortality was infinitely less than in Ceylon where we cannot be said to have a cold season . . ."[310]

The level of mortality quoted by Christie was much higher than equivalent mortality rates in England at about the same time; for example, of the 3,000 people variolated at the London Smallpox Hospital in 1806, only two died.[311] The mortality rates in Ceylon and India may have been inflated by people catching natural smallpox before being variolated, but this also happened as we saw earlier in the London Smallpox Hospital, and is not likely to be able to explain the scale of difference in the success rate of the two series of inoculations. The minimal mortality associated with itinerant Brahmin inoculators was probably not only a function of their variolating in the cold season, but also possibly as a result of their practice of cold water treatment, as well as using virus from previous sites of inoculation.

The historical evidence quoted all more or less relates to the effect of lower temperatures on the outcome of orthodox variolation, but although this has no direct bearing on the attenuating effect of arm-to-arm inoculation, there is a logical relationship at the hypothetical level. It can be shown that there is a significant difference in the average temperature of the skin and inner body areas,[312] and it is probable that the distribution of smallpox lesions on the body, is a function of temperature sensitivity of the virus.[313] Any method of further reducing skin temperature would increase the likelihood of producing cold variants by ensuring that virus was grown at the pustular stage at reduced temperatures. Virus taken from ordinary pustules in orthodox variolation would, of course, have experienced the higher temperatures during the phase of inner-body growth, but this could explain the greater severity of conventional smallpox inoculation over the more attenuated form achieved through arm-to-arm variolation. Virus in the latter procedure would, of course, be systematically selected from the sites of injection in the skin, and would therefore be consistently exposed to the lower body surface temperatures. If one thinks of the ten generations of arm-to-arm inoculation recommended by Thiele in his attenuating procedures, one comes very near to the type of serial passage described by Kirn and Braunwald in the production of the vaccinia cold variant. Although the foregoing argument is purely hypothetical, at least a part of it should be testable in the laboratory. If variola virus taken from pustules or smallpox crusts is different in its characteristics due to a partially different temperature environment, it should display a differential sensitivity to temperature than virus taken from the blood or other inner-body areas. As far as I am aware, no systematic comparison of the temperature characteristics of the two types of virus has ever been undertaken.

What are the overall implications of the findings of this book? As virtually all forms of vaccination during the first forty years of the nineteenth century were attenuated forms of smallpox, the conventional dichotomy between unsafe, dangerous and ineffective variolation on the one hand, and medically sound, safe and effective vaccination on the other, no longer remains valid. Variolation and vaccination should be viewed as a part of a continuum, with the former being more severe in its effects than the latter. Although it might still be argued that variolation did occasionally spread smallpox through respiratory infection — and there can be no doubt about this from the evidence of the Petworth and Marblehead incidents alone — it had the advantage of conferring a much longer period of immunity against natural attacks of smallpox than did the more attenuated vaccination. Once variolation begins to be viewed as only a variation and a more severe form of vaccination, a revision of its historical importance becomes possible. It was always very much less dangerous than conventional medical historical accounts have accused it of being; it is not possible to discuss the historical evidence for this view here, but it might be appropriate to quote from Imperato's recent (1968 and 1974) account of variolation among the Songhai of Mali, to conclude the argument. According to Imperato, out of a total of 120 people variolated in 1967, none died, and only 22 developed a severe enough reaction to be thought to have had "clinical smallpox" (all these cases were "mild, characterised by a rash composed of discrete lesions"). Even these cases, Imperato believed, were likely to have been due to prior infection from natural smallpox during an epidemic. He has described the variolations as follows:

> ". . . the variolation technique used consisted of the application of vesicular fluid with either a thorn or a bird feather to a small round area of 5mm. diameter on the deltoid area of the arm or the lateral aspect of the leg just below

> the knee. There was very little tissue destruction associated with this technique and the inoculum was small . . . The variolation sites did not show any signs of secondary infection . . . According to one infirmier who had rendered medical care to both villages during the epidemic, the sequence of events of the variolation reaction was not unlike that of a normal primary vaccinal reaction. He was aware of only two instances in which satellite lesions appeared around the variolation site. Unfortunately, data could not be obtained about systematic reactions; four men in the village of Lellehoi, who had variolation scars on their right deltoid areas, indistinguishable from vaccination scars, denied any systematic reactions."[314]

It is not surprising that as only 18.3 per cent of the total cases had reactions resembling clinical smallpox (and many of these probably due to natural infection), as few as 7.1 per cent of 447 informants interviewed in a survey said that they believed that the variolation reaction could cause smallpox in others (and those were young people, subjected to the belief patterns of modern medicine). Although Imperato himself implies that this reflects an ignorance of concepts of modern disease, recent work in India has shown that the infectivity of variola virus is partly a function of its virulence,[315] and therefore the very mild cases described by Imperato would probably have very low degrees of infectivity, possibly to the point of being non-infectious. This is not to say that all forms of variolation were as safe as those described above; Imperato also describes other types of variolation using other techniques, which were more dangerous to those being inoculated, and probably to those exposed to possible respiratory infection emanating from them. The safety and nature of variolation varied very significantly depending on the technique and method of inoculation adopted.

CONCLUSION

The evidence discussed in this book points to the conclusion that the bulk of the vaccine used by Jenner and his contemporaries was not derived from cowpox, but was accidentally developed from an attenuated strain of smallpox virus. It might be asked why medical workers and historians have not previously discovered this. Those who investigated the subject in any detail (such as Creighton and Crookshank) did uncover much of the relevant information, but were unable to reach appropriate conclusions because of their involvement in practical disputes about the value of vaccination and their limited scientific understanding of the subject. The heroism with which medical history has portrayed Jenner has all the hallmarks of a medical myth, although some might prefer to see it as one of Kuhn's paradigms of science. The final judgment on the status of Jenner's contribution to medicine must be left to the historians of science, but we may conclude here that his contribution to the control and eventual elimination of smallpox, was only a part — although a very important part — of a long history of smallpox prophylaxsis, which includes both variolation and vaccination, stretching over hundreds, and perhaps even thousands of years.

REFERENCES

1. George Pearson, 'A Letter Concerning a Report of Two Persons Having Died Under the Cow-Pock Inoculation', *The Medical and Physical Journal,* 3 (1800), p. 412.
2. John Ring, *A Treatise on the Cowpox* (1800–03), p. 91.
3. John Baron, *The Life of Edward Jenner,* Vol. I (1838), p. 342.
4. Edward Jenner, *An Inquiry Into The Causes and Effects of the Variolae Vaccinae,* (1798), pp. 32–34.
5. *Ibid.,* pp. 36–42.
6. *Ibid.,* p. 39.
7. *Ibid.,* p. 41.
8. See E. M. Crookshank, *History and Pathology of Vaccination,* Vol. 2 (1889), p. 31, Fn. 14.
9. Baron, *op. cit.,* pp. 150–153.
10. Edward Jenner, *Further Observations on the Variolae Vaccinae Or Cow-Pox,* (1799), pp. 28, 29, 40. Baron, *op. cit.,* p. 308.
11. Jenner, *Further Observations,* pp. 29–31.
12. *Ibid.,* pp. 33, 34.
13. Baron, *op. cit.,* p. 315.
14. "Letter from Mr. Hughes to Jenner", *Medical and Physical Journal,* Vol. I (1799), p. 319; Jenner, *Further Observations,* p. 30.
15. "Letter from Mr. Hughes", *op. cit.,* pp. 319, 320.
16. "Letter from Mr. Thornton, Surgeon, Stroud, Feb. 7, 1799" in Thomas Beddoes (Ed.) *Contributions to Physical and Medical Knowledge* (1799), p. 401.
17. "Letter from Mr. Hughes", *op. cit.,* p. 322.
18. Henry Hicks, *Observations On A Report . . . On . . . Vaccinia* (1803), p. 71.
19. "Letter from Mr. Thornton", *op. cit.,* pp. 399–402.
20. Baron, *op cit.,* p. 309.
21. Jenner, *Further Observations,* p. 39.
22. Jenner, *An Inquiry,* p. 34; Crookshank, *op. cit.,* p. 25.
23. Baron, *op. cit.,* p. 140.
24. Edward Jenner, *A Continuation of Facts and Observa-*

tions Relative To The Variolae Vaccinae Or Cowpox (1800), p. 7.

25. J. B. Estlin, "Second Letter", *The Medical Gazette,* New Series, Vol. I (1838–39), in Crookshank, *op. cit.,* p. 332.
26. R. Ceely, "Observations On The Variolae Vaccinae", *Transactions of the Provincial Medical and Surgical Association,* Vol. 8 (1840), in Crookshank, *op. cit.,* p. 400.
27. *Ibid.,* p. 402.
28. M. Bousquet, *On Cow Pox Discovered At Passy* (1836), in Crookshank, *op. cit.,* p. 321.
29. Baron, *op. cit.,* pp. 307, 308.
30. See for example *Philosophical Transactions,* Vol. 50 (1758), pp. 528–538 and Vol. 70 (1780), pp. 536–548.
31. See for example E. M. Crookshank, *History and Pathology of Vaccination,* Vol. 1 (1889), pp. 298–304.
32. William Woodville, *Reports Of A Series Of Inoculations For The Variolae Vaccinae Or Cowpox,* (1799), pp. 137, 138.
33. *The Report On The . . . Vaccine Pock Institution* (1803), p. 39; Robert Willan, *On Vaccine Inoculation* (1806), pp. 4, 5.
34. Jenner, *An Inquiry,* pp. 4–6, 67.
35. R. Ceely, "Further Observations On The Variolae Vaccinae", *Transactions of the Provincial Medical and Surgical Association,* Vol. X (1842) in Crookshank, *op. cit.,* Vol. 2 (1889).
36. Ceely, "Observations" in Crookshank, *op. cit.,* Vol. 2 (1889), pp. 444-446
37. *Ibid.,* pp. 389, 405.
38. *Ibid.,* p. 389.
39. *Ibid.*
40. Woodville, *Reports,* p. 138.
41. Robert Willan, *On Vaccine Inoculation* (1806), pp. 3–5.
42. Woodville, *Reports,* pp. 37–52.
43. *Ibid.,* p. 137.
44. William Woodville, *Observations On The Cow-Pox* (1800), p. 19.

45. Woodville, *Reports,* pp. 18–34.
46. John Andrew, *The Practice of Inoculation Impartially Considered* (1765), p. 14; Thomas Dimsdale, *The Present Method of Inoculating For The Small-Pox* (1767), pp. 32–33; C. W. Dixon, *Smallpox* (1962), p. 110.
47. Woodville, *Reports,* p. 16.
48. Dixon, *op. cit.,* p. 24.
49. Ring, *op. cit.,* p. 606.
50. Willan, *op. cit.,* p. 8.
51. Woodville, *Reports,* pp. 155, 156.
52. Ring, *op. cit.,* pp. 143, 144.
53. Baron, *op. cit.,* pp. 313, 314; Woodville, *Reports,* p. 141.
54. Woodville, *Reports,* pp. 27–56.
55. *Ibid.,* pp. 25–29.
56. Woodville, *Reports,* pp. 37–46.
57. *Ibid., p.* 16; Dimsdale, *op. cit.,* pp. 32–33; Dixon, *op. cit.,* p. 110.
58. Woodville, *Reports,* pp. 51, 52.
59. *Ibid.,* pp. 54, 55.
60. *Ibid.,* pp. 49, 50.
61. *Ibid.,* pp. 50, 51.
62. *Ibid.,* pp. 55, 56.
63. Baron, *op. cit.,* pp. 316, 317.
64. *Ibid.,* p. 316.
65. *Ibid.,* p. 324.
66. Jenner, *Further Observations,* pp. 56–58.
67. Jenner, *Further Observations,* p. 62.
68. Woodville, *Observations,* p. 11.
69. Baron, *op. cit.,* pp. 316, 317.
70. Jenner, *Further Observations,* pp. 56–59.
71. Baron, *op. cit.,* pp. 324, 325.
72. *Ibid.,* p. 324.
73. *Ibid.,* pp. 322, 323.
74. *Ibid.,* p. 323.
75. Jenner, *Further Observations,* p. 62.
76. Baron, *op. cit.,* p. 379.
77. See Letter from Thomas Tanner to the Royal College of

Physicians in the *Royal College of Physicians Library,* M.S.52.c.15 (9th February, 1807).

78. Ring, *op. cit.,* pp. 27, 647, 649.
79. Jenner, *A Continuation,* pp. 11–12.
80. Baron, *op. cit.,* p. 357.
81. *Ibid.,* p. 325.
82. Woodville, *Observations,* p. 11.
83. Jenner, *A Continuation,* p. 19.
84. Baron, *op. cit.,* p. 356.
85. Genevieve Miller, "Letters of Edward Jenner", *Medical Arts and Sciences,* Vol. 2, No. 1 (1948), p. 12.
86. Jenner, *A Continuation,* p. 22.
87. *Ibid.,* p. 6.
88. Baron, *op. cit.,* pp. 348, 349.
89. See dedication to Edward Jenner, *A Continuation of Facts and Observations Relative To The Variolae Vaccinae* bound with the second edition of his *Inquiry* and *Further Observations,* (1800).
90. Baron, *op. cit.,* p. 343.
91. See *Further Observations,* pp. 56–60.
92. Miller, *op. cit.,* p. 12.
93. *Ibid.,* p. 358.
94. Baron, *op. cit.,* p. 357.
95. Ring, *op. cit.,* p. 636.
96. *Ibid.,* pp. 27, 647.
97. *Ibid.,* p. 458.
98. Benjamin Waterhouse, *A Prospect of Exterminating The Small Pox,* Part 2 (1802), pp. 110–116.
99. *Ibid.,* p. 21.
100. "Jenner's Evidence, 19th February, 1807", *Royal College of Physicians Vaccination Committee* (M.S. 1928/326), p. 31.
101. "Letter from John Ring, 15th January, 1802", *Medical and Physical Journal,* 7 (1802), pp. 109–110.
102. "Letter from J. De Carro to Dr. A. Munro, Vienna, 13th July, 1825", *Medical and Physical Journal,* I (1826), pp. 284, 285.
103. "Jenner's Evidence, 19th February, 1807", *op. cit.,* p. 36.

104. E. M. Crookshank, *History and Pathology of Vaccination,* Vol. I (1889), p. 390.
105. John Baron, *The Life of Edward Jenner,* Vol. 2 (1838), p. 398.
106. Miller, *op. cit.,* p. 16.
107. Baron, *op. cit.,* Vol. 2, pp. 226, 418; Baron, *op. cit.,* Vol. 1, p. 254.
108. Baron, *op. cit.,* Vol. 1, p. 254; Baron, *op. cit.,* Vol. 2, p. 226.
109. "Report of the National Vaccine Establishment", *Medical Gazette,* II (1838), p. 349.
110. "Report of the National Vaccine Establishment, January, 1840", in Crookshank, *op. cit.,* Vol. 2, p. 530.
111. See C. R. Aikin, "Renewal of the Vaccine Virus", *Medical Gazette,* (1840), p. 190.
112. See Woodville, *Reports* for the evidence on which the following statistics in the text are derived.
113. William Watson, *An Account of a Series of Experiments . . . of Inoculating Smallpox* (1768), p. 24.
114. Woodville, *Reports,* p. 62.
115. *Ibid.,* pp. 151–155.
116. *Ibid.,* p. 152.
117. "Letter from W. Woodville", *The Medical and Physical Journal,* July, 1799, Vol. I, p. 417.
118. G. C. Jenner, *The Evidence at Large . . .* (1805), p. 25.
119. "Letter from W. Woodville", *op. cit.,* p. 417.
120. Woodville, *Observations,* p. 40.
121. "Letter from W. Woodville, December 1800", *Medical and Physical Journal,* 3, (1800), p. 36.
122. G. C. Jenner, *op. cit.,* p. 25.
123. John Adams, *A Popular View of Vaccine Inoculation* (1807), pp. 130, 131.
124. Woodville, *Observations,* p. 21.
125. Woodville, *Reports,* pp. 141, 142.
126. Woodville, *Observations,* p. 22.
127. Ring, *A Treatise,* p. 301.
128. George Pearson, *An Examination of the Report on the Committee of the House of Commons* (1802), p. 44.
129. *Ibid.,* p. 108.

130. G. C. Jenner, *op. cit.*, p. 133.
131. Pearson, *An Examination*, p. 45.
132. Ring, *A Treatise*, p. 302.
133. George Pearson, "A Communication Concerning The Eruptions Resembling The Small-Pox, Which Sometimes Appear In The Inoculated Vaccine Disease", *Medical and Physical Journal*, Vol. 3, Feb. 1800, p. 99.
134. George Pearson, "On The Present State Of The Evidence With Regard To The Vaccine Inoculation", *Medical and Physical Journal*, Vol. 3 (1800), p. 399.
135. Baron, *op. cit.*, Vol. I, pp. 313, 314. See also Pearson, "A Communication . . ." *op. cit.*, p. 98.
136. Pearson, *An Examination*, p. 45.
137. *Ibid.*, p. 55.
138. Pearson, *A Communication*, p. 98.
139. *Ibid.*, p. 99.
140. *Ibid.*, p. 99.
141. *Ibid.*, p. 100.
142. Pearson, *An Examination*, p. 155.
143. *The Report on the . . . Vaccine-Pock Institution* (1803), p. 17.
144. Pearson, *An Examination*, p. 155.
145. Jenner, *A Continuation*, p. 22.
146. *The Report on the . . . Vaccine-Pock Institution* (1803), p. 17.
147. "Report on the Cow-Pock Inoculation, from the practice at the Vaccine-Pock Institution, during the years 1800, 1801 and 1802", *Medical and Chirurigical Review*, 10 (1803–04), pp. 50, 51.
148. *Ibid.*, p. 53.
149. James Moore, *The History and Practice of Vaccination* (1817), p. 31.
150. "Letter from the Rev. Robert Holt of Finmere, 6th November, 1799", *Medical and Physical Journal*, 2 (1799), p. 403; and Woodville, *Observations*, p. 17.
151. *Letter from Dr. Walker of Leeds to Lettsom, 9th October, 1801* (Letter Number 16486, Wellcome Institute History Library).
152. "Letters from J. Evans of Ketley, Shropshire to W.

Woodville, 11th and 29th September, 1799", *Medical and Physical Journal,* 2 (1799), pp. 310, 311, 312.
153. Dr. R. Redfearn "Three Cases of Inoculation with the Variolae Vaccinae", *Medical and Physical Journal,* 2 (1799), pp. 23–25.
154. Ring, *A Treatise,* p. 394; Baron, *op. cit.,* Vol. I, p. 378.
155. "Letter from Dr. J. W. Barry to G. Pearson, 1st October, 1800", *Medical and Physical Journal,* 4 (1800), p. 428.
156. "Mr. Stromeyer's Letter Concerning The Vaccine Inoculation Practised By Him", *Medical and Physical Journal,* 3 (1800), p. 473.
157. H. M. Husson, "Reserches Historiques Et Medicales" in *Recuil de Memoires D'Observations et Experiences* (1801), p. 54.
158. "On Vaccine Inoculation in Rotterdam", *Medical and Physical Journal,* 7 (1802), pp. 251–256.
159. Baron, *op. cit.,* Vol. I, pp. 327–329.
160. *Letter to Dr. John Walker, Royal Jennerian Society, 25th January, 1805 from the Vaccine Institute, Edinburgh Dispensary* (Wellcome Institute for the History of Medicine Library).
161. "Letter from W. Simmons on Vaccine", *Medical and Physical Journal* 5, (1801), p. 135.
162. "Letter from J. H. Grosse, Winslow, 15th March, 1800", *Medical and Physical Journal,* 3 (1800), p. 295; "Letter from J. H. Grosse, Winslow, 6th April, 1801", *Medical and Physical Journal,* 5 (1801), p. 453.
163. Ring, *A Treatise,* p. 491.
164. *Ibid.,* p. 523.
165. "Letter from Dr. D. Paterson, Montrose, 25th May, 1801", *Medical and Physical Journal,* 6 (1801), pp. 42, 43.
166. Joseph Adams, *Some Account of . . . the Hospital for Small-Pox Inoculation . . . and for Vaccination* (1817), p. 15.
167. "Letter from T. K. Kelson, Seven Oaks, May 19th, 1800", *Medical and Physical Journal,* 4 (1800), p. 22.
168. Redfearn, *op. cit.,* pp. 23–25.
169. "Letter from Dr. Walker, *op. cit.*

170. "Letter from the Rev. Robert Holt", *op. cit.*, p. 403.
171. "Letter from the Rev. W. Finch, 11th March, 1800, *Medical and Physical Journal,* 3 (1800), pp. 415–418.
172. "Letter from M. Ward, Manchester, 12th July, 1799, *Medical and Physical Journal,* 2 (1799), p. 134.
173. "Letter from W. Simmons on Vaccine", 9th December, 1800, *Medical and Physical Journal,* 5 (1801), p. 135. The Vaccine Institute attached to the Edinburgh Dispensary seems to have had a similar experience, but they attempted to explain these frequent cases of pustular eruption as being due to chicken-pox. See *Letter . . . from the Vaccine Institute, Edinburgh Dispensary, op. cit.*
174. See Crookshank, *op. cit.*, Vol. 2, p. 184 (see especially footnote); Baron, *op. cit.*, Vol. I, p. 152.
175. Baron, *op. cit.*, Vol. I, pp. 358, 359.
176. Miller, *op. cit.*, p. 12.
177. *Ibid.*
178. Baron, *op. cit.*, Vol. I, p. 344.
179. Jenner, *A Continuation,* p. 10 Fn.
180. *Ibid.*, pp. 21, 22.
181. "Letter from Edward Jenner, 13th January, 1800", *Medical and Physical Journal,* Vol. 3 (1800), p. 102.
182. "Letter from Edward Jenner, 15th May, 1800", *Medical and Physical Journal,* Vol. 3 (1800), p. 502.
183. Waterhouse, *op. cit.*, p. 115.
184. Evidence of Jenner, 19th February, 1807, *Royal College of Physicians Vaccination Committee Minute Book,* (MS 1928/326).
185. Jenner, *Further Observations,* p. 14.
186. *Ibid.*, p. 18.
187. "Letters from J. Evans of Ketley, Shropshire to W. Woodville", 11th September and 29th September, *Medical and Physical Journal,* 2, (1799), p. 311.
188. *Ibid.*, pp. 311, 312.
189. *Ibid.*, p. 312.
190. *Ibid.*, p. 312.
191. *Ibid.*, pp. 311, 312.
192. Pearson, "On the Present State . . ." *op. cit.*, p. 401.

193. "Letter from John Ring, M.D., 6th May, 1800", *London Medical Review and Magazine,* 3 (1800), p. 314.
194. Ring, *A Treatise,* pp. 636, 637.
195. "Letter from John Ring", *op. cit.,* p. 314.
196. "Translation of Mr. Stromeyer's letter Concerning the Vaccine Inoculation Practised by Him", *Medical and Physical Journal,* 3, (1800), p. 472.
197. Baron, *op. cit.,* Vol. I, pp. 381, 382.
198. R. J. Thornton, *Facts in Favour of the Cow-Pock* (1803), pp. 192, 193, 198, 209, 210.
199. *Ibid.,* p. 230.
200. "Letter from J. Blount to Jenner, 14th June, 1801", *Medical and Physical Journal,* 6 (1801), p. 115.
201. Baron, *op. cit.,* Vol. I, p. 386. See also Waterhouse, *op. cit.,* p. 113.
202. Waterhouse, *op. cit.,* pp. 5, 23, 24.
203. Ring, *A Treatise,* p. 755.
204. Benjamin Waterhouse, *A Prospect of Exterminating the Small-Pox,* Part I (1800), p. 21.
205. *Ibid.,* pp. 23, 24.
206. Ring, *A Treatise,* p. 756.
207. *Ibid.,* p. 755.
208. Waterhouse, *A Prospect, Part II,* p. 15.
209. Morris C. Leikind, "An Episode in the History of Small-pox Vaccination in New Hampshire", *John Hopkins Institute History of Medicine Bulletin,* VII (1939), pp. 676, 677.
210. *Ibid.,* p. 678.
211. John B. Blake, *Benjamin Waterhouse and the Introduction of Vaccination* (1957), p. 25.
212. "Letter from Waterhouse, 14th November, 1800", *Columbian Sentinel,* 19th November, 1800.
213. "Letter from 'Anti-Synopsis', 15th December, 1800", reprinted in *The Independent Chronicle,* 1st–5th January, 1801.
214. "Letter from Waterhouse, 20th December, 1800", *Columbian Sentinel,* 27th December, 1800.
215. Waterhouse, *A Prospect, Part 2,* p. 10.
216. "Letter from Waterhouse, 14th November, 1800", *op.*

cit.; Waterhouse, *A Prospect, Part 2,* p. 10.

217. Waterhouse, *A Prospect, Part 2,* p. 7.
218. See *The Medical and Physical Journal,* 6 (1801), pp. 326, 327.
219. Waterhouse, *A Prospect, Part 2,* pp. 14, 15.
220. *Ibid.,* pp. 17, 18.
221. *Ibid.,* p. 9.
222. *Ibid.,* p. 118.
223. *Ibid.,* p. 13.
224. *Ibid.,* p. 9.
225. *Ibid.,* p. 10.
226. *"Letter From Elisha Story to the Massachusetts Medical Society, 4 May, 1801* (In the Francis Countway Library of Medicine, Boston).
227. *Columbian Sentinel,* 14th January, 1801.
228. William Bentley, *The Diary of William Bentley, D.D.* (1907), p. 355.
229. *Ibid.,* p. 357.
230. *Ibid.,* p. 356.
231. *Ibid.,* p. 357.
232. "Letter from Waterhouse", *The Columbian Sentinel,* 19th April, 1806.
233. "Letter from Waterhouse", 16th July, 1806, *The Columbian Sentinel,* 23rd July, 1806.
234. Ring, *A Treatise,* p. 458.
235. Waterhouse, *A Prospect, Part 2,* pp. 110–116.
236. *Ibid.,* p. 33.
237. *Ibid.,* p. 67.
238. *Ibid.,* p. 112.
239. Baron, *op. cit.,* Vol. I, p. 389.
240. H. M. Husson, "Reserches Historiques et Medicales", in *Recuil de Memoires D'Observations et Experiences,* (1801), p. 52.
241. *Ibid.,* pp. 40, 41, 42, 48.
242. *Ibid.,* p. 53.
243. *Ibid.,* p. 54, *Royal Commission on Vaccination, 6th Report,* p. 309.
244. Husson, *op. cit.,* p. 98.
245. *Ibid.,* p. 53.

246. *Ibid.*, p. 53.
247. Baron, *op. cit.*, Vol. I, p. 440.
248. Ring, *A Treatise*, p. 409.
249. *Ibid.*, pp. 426, 427.
250. "Letter from Jenner to Dr. Marcet, 23rd February, 1803", *Medical and Physical Journal*, 9 (1803), pp. 462–464.
251. Baron, *op. cit.*, Vol. I, pp. 450, 474, 475.
252. *Ibid.*. p. 476.
253. "Letter from Jenner to Marcet", *op. cit.*, pp. 2–4.
254. George Gregory, *Lectures on the Eruptive Fevers* (1843), p. 187.
255. Charles Creighton, *The Natural History of Cow-Pox* (1887), p. 92.
256. Edward Ballard, *On Vaccination* (1868), p. 224.
257. "Letter from J. De Carro to Dr. A. Monro, Vienna, July 13th, 1825", *The Edinburgh Journal of Medical Science*, Vol. 1 (1826), p. 284.
258. Ballard, *op. cit.*, pp. 216–234.
259. James Moore, *The History and Practice of Vaccination* (1817), p. 36.
260. J. Z. Holwell, *An Account of the Manner of Inoculating for the Smallpox on the East Indies* (1767), pp. 17, 20.
261. Angelo Gatti, *New Observations on Inoculation* (1768), p. 39, fn. a.
262. Dr. Giles Watts, *A Vindication of the New Method of Inoculating the Smallpox* (1767), p. 23; Dr. George Baker, *An Inquiry into the Merits of a Method of Inoculating the Small-Pox* (1766), p. 9; B. Chandler, *An Essay Towards an Investigation . . . of Inoculation* (1767), p. 7; Thomas Dimsdale, *The Present Method of Inoculating for the Small-Pox* (1767), p. 27.
263. Watts, *op. cit.*, p. 23; Dimsdale, *op. cit.*, p. 26.
264. R. Houlton, *Indisputable Facts Relative to the Suttonian Art of Inoculation* (1768), p. 40.
265. Watts, *op. cit.*, p. 39.
266. William Bromfield, *Thoughts Arising from Experience Concerning . . . the Small-Pox* (1767), pp. 10, 11.

267. J. Mudge, *A Dissertation on the Inoculated Smallpox* (1777), pp. 20–22.
268. *Ibid.*, p. 23.
269. John Covey, "Further Observations and Facts Relative to the Practice of Inoculation of the Small-Pox", *The London Medical Journal,* 1787, pp. 6, 7.
270. Dimsdale, *op. cit.*, p. 26.
271. Chandler, *op. cit.*, p. 30.
272. C. Salmade, *Instruction sur la Pratique de L'Inoculation de la Petite Verole* (1799), pp. 51, 52.
273. Joseph Adams, *A Popular View of Vaccine Inoculation* (1807), p. 27.
274. Crookshank, *op. cit.*, Vol. I, pp. 289, 290.
275. Adams, *A Popular View,* p. 156.
276. *Ibid.*, p. 158.
277. Crookshank, *op. cit.*, Vol. I, p. 291.
278. Adams, *A Popular View,* pp. v, vi.
279. *Ibid.*, p. 158.
280. Baron, *op. cit.*, Vol. I, p. 246.
281. *Ibid.*
282. M. Guillon, "Experiments upon the Inoculation of Smallpox", *Medical and Foreign Review,* IV, No. 23 (1827), p. 426.
283. Dr. Basil Thiele, "Smallpox and Cowpox , Their Identity, and the Reverting of the Former to Vaccine", *Henke's Journal,* No. 1 (Erlangen, 1839), p. 7.
284. *Ibid.*, p. 3.
285. *Ibid.*, pp. 10, 11, 19, 20.
286. A. Trousseau, *Clinical Medicine,* 2 (1869), pp. 91–93.
287. *Ibid.*, p. 92.
288. A. W. Downie, "Smallpox", in Stuart Mudd (Ed.), *Infectious Agents and Host Reactions* (1970); Dixon, *op. cit.*
289. See A. Herrlich et al., "Experimental Studies on Transformation of the Variola Virus into the Vaccinia Virus", *Archiv Fur Die Gesamte Virusforschung,* 12 (1963), p. 596.
290. *Ibid.*, for a review of the evidence.

291. *Ibid.*
292. See S. Monckton Copeman, *Vaccination: Its Natural History and Pathology* (1899), pp. 60, 63; E. S. Horgan, "The Experimental Transformation of Variola to Vaccinia", *The Journal of Hygiene,* 38 (1938).
293. Crookshank, *op. cit.,* Vol. 2, p. 520.
294. Copeman, *op. cit.,* p. 47.
295. *Ibid.*
296. H. S. Bedson and K. R. Dumbell, "Variola Major and Cowpox Hybrids", *The Journal of Hygiene* (Cambridge), 62 (1964), p. 157; Herrlich, *op. cit.,* p. 596.
297. Crookshank, *op. cit.,* Vol. 2, pp. 326–332, 399–403; Copeman, *op. cit.,* p. 71.
298. J. A. Dudgeon, "Development of Smallpox Vaccine in England in the Eighteenth and Nineteenth Centuries", *British Medical Journal* (May, 1963), p. 1371.
299. J. C. G. Ledingham and D. McClean, "The Propagation of Vaccine Virus in the Rabbit Dermis", *British Journal of Experimental Pathology",* Vol. 9 (1928), pp. 218–224.
300. Personal communication from Professor Keith Dumbell, St. Mary's Hospital.
301. Baxby, *op. cit.,* p. 223.
302. Derrick Baxby, "A Possible Relation between Human Patogenicity of Smallpox Vaccines and Virus Growth at Elevated Temperatures", *Journal of Hygiene* (Cambridge), 73, 1974.
303. A. Kirn and J. Braunwald, "The Selection of a 'Cold' Variant with a Weaker Virulence than the Vaccinial Virus, By Transfers at Low Temperatures", *Annales de l'Institut Pasteur,* 106 (1964), p. 437.
304. *Ibid.,* p. 438.
305. A. H. Griffith "Viral Vaccines" in J. E. Banatvala (Ed), *Current Problems in Chemical Virology* (1971), p. 154.
306. Holwell, *op. cit.,* p. 18.
307. Gatti, *op. cit.,* p. 68.
308. K. Dewhurst (Ed), *Dr. Thomas Sydenham,* 1624–89 (1966), p. 106.
309. See Dimsdale, *op. cit.,* pp. 6, 7.

310. Thomas Christie, *An Account of the Ravages Committed in Ceylon by Small-Pox Previously to the Introduction of Vaccination* (1811), pp. 15, 16. See also James Bryce, *Practical Observations on Cowpox* (1809), p. 8 for confirmation of this evidence.

311. Adams, *A Popular View, op. cit.*, p. 56.

312. George H. Bell, *Textbook of Physiology and Biochemistry* (1965), p. 865.

313. Downie, in Mudd, *op. cit.*, p. 504.

314. P. J. Imperato, "The Practice of Variolation among the Songhai of Mali", *Transactions of the Royal Society of Tropical Medicine and Hygiene,* 62 (1968); P. J. Imperato, "Observations on Variolation Practices in Mali", *Tropical and Geographical Medicine,* 26 (1974). For a similar recent favourable account of variolation, see C. D. Rosenwald, "Variolation and other observations during a smallpox epidemic in the Southern Province of Tanganyika", *The Medical Officer,* March, 1951.

315. J. K. Sarkar et al., "Virus Excretion in Smallpox", *Bulletin of the World Health Organisation,* 48, (1973), pp. 517–522.

INDEX